THE BOWEL CANCER RECOVERY TOOLKIT

GET WELL FASTER WITH ACTIVITY, EXERCISE AND LIFESTYLE

This book is dedicated to you, the reader.

I hope it provides you with knowledge, courage and inspiration.

THE BOWEL CANCER RECOVERY TOOLKIT

GET WELL FASTER WITH ACTIVITY, EXERCISE AND LIFESTYLE

Sarah Russell

Foreword by Dr Juliet McGrattan

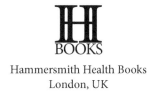

BOOKS

Hammersmith Health Books
London, UK

First published in 2019 by Hammersmith Health Books – an imprint of Hammersmith Books Limited
4/4A Bloomsbury Square, London WC1 2RP, UK
www.hammersmithbooks.co.uk

Reprinted 2019, 2021 (revised), 2022 (revised)

British Library Cataloguing in Publication Data: A CIP record of this book is available from the British Library.

Print ISBN 978-1-78161-136-4
Ebook ISBN 978-1-78161-137-1

Commissioning editor: Georgina Bentliff
Edited by: Carolyn White
Designed and typeset by: Julie Bennett, Bespoke Publishing Ltd.
Cover design by: Sylvia Kwan
Cover illustration © KN; SpicyTruffel / shutterstock.com
Index: Dr Laurence Errington
Production: Helen Whitehorn, Path Projects Ltd.
Printed and bound by: TJ Books Limited, Cornwall, UK

Contents

Foreword

Dr Juliet McGrattan
Author of *Sorted: The Active Woman's Guide to Health* and former GP

Working as a GP I would see many patients go from being diagnosed with bowel cancer to then progressing through treatment. It's an incredibly stressful and worrying time when people can feel vulnerable and disempowered. Suddenly the everyday becomes medicalised in what can seem like a constant stream of hospital appointments and medication. There's a tendency to think that rest is best to help you cope with all this, but we now know that the reverse is often true. Being active can help improve survival rates for colorectal cancer, reduce the risk of cancer recurring, speed up recovery and also improve tolerance to treatment by helping to reduce side-effects. Exercise is something that people with cancer can use in a positive way to help them feel more relaxed and in control at this challenging time.

It is not easy to exercise during cancer treatment, but it is important, and the benefits are significant. Patients tend to assume that doing exercise will just tire them out more but actually an activity like brisk walking can help to reduce the fatigue and general weakness commonly caused by cancer and chemotherapy treatment. Moving around also helps to maintain muscle strength which can be quickly lost with inactivity; this is particularly important after surgery. Exercise has been found to increase the number and activity of natural killer cells which the body makes to try to destroy cancer cells. It also triggers the release of myokines from muscles; these act as anti-inflammatories which help to prevent and treat cancer. I would make sure that my patients knew that keeping as fit as they could was part of their treatment and would help them to make a faster recovery as well as helping them through the treatment itself.

I found I needed to reassure people that they might not be anywhere near their usual exercise levels, particularly if they were previously very active, but that didn't matter; this is definitely a situation where doing something is better than doing nothing. Even a short walk in the fresh air can be enough to give you a little boost of energy. Don't forget that exercise causes the release of endorphins in the body; these help to relax you and lift your mood and can help to reduce pain too – three very important reasons why cancer and exercise are a good combination.

Exercise is important for all of us, but it has a particular importance when you're going through treatment for colorectal cancer. It can feel like the toughest time to be active, but if you take it slowly and gradually you will see that the benefits are worth the effort. Taking control of this aspect of your treatment is something to be very proud of.

Testimonials

Dr Lucy Gossage
Oncologist, professional triathlete and co-founder of www.cancerfit.me

Every couple of weeks I get an email or message on social media from someone newly diagnosed with bowel cancer or recovering from cancer treatment, asking me how they can stay active during their treatment or regain fitness after treatment. The evidence is clear. Exercise before, during and after treatment has numerous benefits, both physical and psychological, for those living with and beyond cancer. However, at the moment, there is very little guidance out there and nowhere for me to refer people for advice. 'Can I keep cycling during my chemo?' 'My doctors have told me no running for 8 weeks – is this true?' 'Does exercise increase my risk of infection during chemo?' 'What can I do with a PICC line?' 'Can I exercise with a stoma?' 'How quickly can I go back to the gym after bowel surgery?' Just some of the questions I get asked on a regular basis, and I am very far from being an expert! Sarah's book is a fantastic starting point for someone living with or beyond colorectal cancer who wants to find out more about exercise during and after cancer treatment. Being active is one of the biggest things you can do to improve your experience and this book will help you achieve that. In addition, we hope that our website www.cancerfit.me will be an additional useful resource, with blogs from patients and experts, and also provide a forum for you to share ideas and concerns with other people aiming to stay active with and after cancer. So, if you're interested in finding out more, please do check it out. Enjoy the read and good luck!

Joan Barker, patient

When I was diagnosed with colorectal cancer in 2017, I, like most people, wanted to be able to reference information about how this would impact me in both the short and long term. At the time of diagnosis, I was as fit and active as I had been in all my life, regularly running, cycling, swimming, playing golf and taking part in running races and triathlons. I was 60 at the time of my diagnosis and, being very honest, my biggest concern wasn't the cancer, it was how would it impact my ability to exercise in the future. Exercise is and has always been key to my health and wellbeing, both physically and mentally. As well as talking to my surgeon, I wanted to be as informed as possible about how to recover well from the surgery and work with my surgeon to ensure the best possible outcome. I wanted to read specifically about how quickly I could exercise after surgery and indeed what specific exercises I could do and when. I was looking for something similar to a training programme to follow (as I had when I was training for the marathon); sadly, I was unable to find anything that would guide me through this process. This was depressing for me as I thought I might end up suddenly only being able to shuffle about my home instead of living at my usual 100-mile-an-hour pace!

I was incredibly lucky to have an amazing stoma nurse and when I expressed my concerns, she explained that it was very important to exercise after surgery, but it had to be the right type of exercise. She then told me that she would put me in touch with an exercise specialist who would guide me through the process. I know I always embarrass Sarah when I say this, but it really is no exaggeration to say that her advice and knowledge prevented me from going into a deep depression. I followed Sarah's advice and was able to swim and take gentle runs only three weeks after surgery. I was confident to run a 5k race whilst having my stoma and continued with her programme after my reversal surgery. My surgeon is thrilled with how quickly I recovered and two years post op I am able to be very active with complete confidence. This book will be an invaluable tool to anyone diagnosed with colorectal cancer and also to their families; part of my battle was reassuring my family that I was actually allowed to exercise! I cannot thank Sarah enough for being there for me; she is an amazing person and a very knowledgeable professional.

Scott Smith, patient

At the age of 28 being told I had colorectal cancer completely shattered my world. Having thoughts wondering if I would ever make it to 30 years old was not something I had expected. My diagnosis was a whirlwind. I had actually been diagnosed with ulcerative colitis initially, but only a few short weeks later was told I had bowel cancer and needed immediate surgery. I had been a moderately heavy smoker, smoking approx. 20–30 cigarettes per day. I had given up smoking to save funds for my wedding and only then did I get symptoms. It seems that the nicotine had caused my colitis to remain undiagnosed for several years. By the time it was discovered it had mutated into bowel cancer.

Thankfully my surgery was relatively routine, which involved having a colectomy (removal of my large intestine) with a permanent stoma. I didn't need chemotherapy or any other treatment. After this life-changing surgery, my life gradually returned to normal, I went back to work, and my wife and I started a family and had our son.

But a few years after my operation my weight gain began to cause me issues with my stoma and leakage with my bag. I also had my son to consider and was finding it hard to keep up with this fast-moving and energetic toddler! So, I decided I would get fit… but I had no idea where to start. I had never been into fitness and had rarely stepped inside a gym.

Through a mutual friend, I was fortunate enough to meet a great personal trainer who tailored my workouts to accommodate the surgery I'd had. He was unable to find any guidance on how to train anyone with a stoma, so instead he developed a training routine that was like one for a new mother after a C-section birth – as it turned out this was the perfect approach. We focused on slowly building my core strength and overall fitness with a mix of gym work, weight training, cardiovascular training and very specific core work. It took time to build my confidence and knowledge of my body – not only did I have a stoma, but I'd never done any exercise before, so knew very little about fitness and movement. I now run regularly and compete in demanding obstacle course races which has changed my life in so many ways.

As I look back, I was fortunate to meet such a great fitness trainer who took the time to understand my medical history and help me build up my confidence and fitness appropriately. However, I am very aware not everyone will be so lucky. I met Sarah Russell some years later and she agreed with the approach of my trainer. I wish I'd known her at the start of my journey. This book will be a great resource for people who aren't as lucky as I was; also, I'm sure, many fitness instructors, nurses and even doctors will find it helpful and informative. If this book had been available to me then it would have given me hope and structure for my recovery. I could have avoided the darker early days of my recovery which I experienced because I had no guidance. Now many years later, exercise has become, for me, less about the obvious physical benefits and more about my psychological fitness. Everyone underestimates how beneficial exercise and activity can be to our mental health. Living with a stoma can be challenging at times and I really believe that exercise can help us cope. In this book, Sarah has developed some fantastic tools and ways in which to rebuild confidence and get active, whether like me you're new to exercise, or if you're getting back into fitness after your surgery. There's something in here for everyone. I wish you well and good luck.

About the author

I'm deeply passionate about exercise and physical activity of any kind. I have devoted my career, and most of my life, to helping others be more active and have a healthy relationship with exercise.

I have a degree and postgraduate Masters in Sport and Exercise Science and I'm a qualified level 4 cancer and exercise rehabilitation specialist and qualified UK athletics running coach with 25 years' experience as an exercise specialist, trainer, coach and health writer. As a 'Clinical Exercise Specialist' I sit somewhere between a physiotherapist and fitness trainer, combining the best of both professions and spanning the gap between exercise and clinical practice.

I believe in 'intuitive exercise', listening to your body and engaging in activity which makes you feel healthy and strong. I believe that exercise should be nourishing and energising – the sort of exercise that makes you feel 'that was nice, I can do that again!' rather than 'I hate it, I ache all over and I'm exhausted'.

For over two decades I have worked with thousands of people using exercise as a therapy to manage a wide range of conditions and needs – heart conditions and stroke, chronic fatigue, injuries, illness and after-surgery, as well as hundreds of injured runners, and more recently, stoma and cancer patients.

Even though I have been into sport my entire life, it took me experiencing serious illness myself to learn just how important exercise is for our health, recovery and mental wellbeing – yet equally just how very difficult it is when we're sick. I have a stoma (ileostomy) myself (see 'My story' in the Appendix) and went through five major bowel surgeries in 18 months. Not because of cancer, so I can't tell you what chemo or radiotherapy are like, but I do know how surgery knocks you off your feet and how challenging it can be to learn to live with a stoma.

I'm in the unique position of being able to combine my professional and personal experience, and now specialise in stoma and bowel cancer rehabilitation and run an exercise consultancy service. I'm recognised as a leading specialist in this specific area and have published research in the *British Journal of Nursing* and presented my work all over the world.

As part of this work, I developed the world's first nurse education programme for global medical devices company ConvaTec (www.convatec.co.uk), for bowel cancer/stoma nurses working in the NHS and private practice. I now train stoma nurses around the world and, in the UK alone, have trained hundreds of NHS stoma nurses, surgeons and physios.

I'm immensely proud of how this work has changed practice for many clinicians and has improved the lives of many patients. Instead of advising patients to rest, these enlightened clinicians are now encouraging stoma and cancer patients to be active during their treatment and recovery.

Ultimately, it's helping people to recover faster with a better long-term outcome, becoming healthier and living an active lifestyle despite their health issues or medical diagnosis.

I have a clinic in East Sussex/Kent where I see clients and offer 1:1 coaching, cancer rehab and biomechanics and I also offer a 'virtual stoma clinic' and mentoring via skype or online.

I'm also privileged to work as a volunteer at The Hospice in the Weald in Kent, where I support the physiotherapy team and deliver weekly exercise groups for patients with advanced disease. I find this work deeply satisfying and it's an honour to be able to work with these patients who benefit so much from being active.

Above all, I'm passionate about helping people develop a healthy relationship with exercise to have in their lives forever.

Find out more about me and my services in the 'My story' section on page 189.

Scan here to go directly to my website (www.sarah-russell.co.uk).

Acknowledgements

Writing this book has been one of the hardest things I've ever done. It's a huge responsibility and privilege to write about such an important topic, and not something I've taken on lightly. My only goal is to try and help people and to support, educate and encourage and to start to change understanding and practice.

The book has taken almost two years from inception to publication and it's an amalgamation of the last eight years of professional practice and personal experience, as well as hundreds of hours of research. I hope I've got the tone, advice and content right.

There are too many people to thank individually, and I'm sorry if I've missed anyone out… but here goes.

Personally, I'd like to thank my family, my mum, husband John and my boys, Edd and Charlie, for their patience, support and encouragement and the frequent 'How's that book coming along?' comments of support … followed by 'Haven't you finished it yet?' I'm sure they're hoping I'll never write another.

Thank you to my best friend Maxine who took a punt on a young 21-year-old sport science graduate back in 1993, gave me my first job and launched my career. Just over 25 years later it's still so much fun to debate the latest exercise science research and trends. And who knew we'd both end up having our own bowel surgery journeys?

Thank you to my publisher, Hammersmith Books, who, when I suggested the topic 'Bowel cancer and exercise' for a book, didn't turn it down, but jumped at the idea with a sense of responsibility and enthusiasm, knowing it was desperately needed. And to my editor Carolyn White for her brutally honest feedback, super-efficient editing and for making the book so much better than it otherwise would have been. Thank you both for waiting patiently whilst I wrote, re-wrote and re-wrote the manuscript.

Thank you to all the wonderful nurses, doctors, surgeons, physios and healthcare professionals around the world that I've had the pleasure to meet and work with over the last few years. I am in awe of what you do – you've taught me so much. I hope that you'll feel this book is a great resource to recommend to your patients.

And personally, I must thank my own surgeon Professor Sina Dorudi at the Princess Grace Hospital, who gave me my life back and who continues to be a huge supporter of what I do and how I live my life. Thank you for listening and treating me like a person, not a patient.

Thank you to Caroline Rudoni, Anette Understup, and the amazing team at ConvaTec, who have been huge advocates from the start. They continue to invest in and support training for nurses and education for patients through me+recovery – the best rehab programme for stoma patients in the world (see page 195).

Thank you to physio Julie Harker and the team at Hospice in the Weald in Kent, who allow me the honour of volunteering and supporting cancer patients with our amazing little exercise groups. It is genuinely one of the greatest and most humbling things I do.

Thank you to Professor Anna Campbell and the team at CanRehab who taught me so much about cancer and exercise and how to deliver a brilliant training course.

And to Dr Juliet McGrattan, Sophie Medlin and Dr Lucy Gossage – you're all amazing and such great role models. Thank you for your support and all you do for patients.

To Joan Barker, who was the inspiration for this project. I looked for a reputable book I could recommend to her, but couldn't find one, so I decided to write it myself. Thank you, Joan, for openly sharing your story with the world and for your ongoing support.

To Scott Smith, you continue to be an inspiration to so many people and your story always brings a tear to my eye. It's never easy talking openly about what we've been through, but you do it with such grace and humility.

To both of you, keep moving, keep sharing and keep doing what you do. You're both superstars.

And to all the other oncology exercise researchers and clinicians around the world. I follow your fabulous research and stalk you on social media and at conferences, and I hope you think I've done a good job with this book. Keep up the great work!

And finally, this book is dedicated to anyone who has ever had bowel cancer. It's never something you think will happen to you and it can be tough and relentless. But I hope you can find a way to include exercise and activity into your life, because I know it will help you.

When I hear from a patient that they're more active because of something I said at a conference or workshop, or that they feel more confident because of doing the exercises I prescribe or that my advice has changed their life, that literally makes my heart sing. It makes it all worthwhile.

And so, to conclude, in the words of Winnie the Pooh:

'There is something you must always remember. You are braver than you believe, stronger than you seem, and smarter than you think.'

Introduction

Bowel cancer (also known as colon or colorectal cancer) is the fourth most common cancer in the UK today (2021) with around 42,000 new cases each year.[1] Treatment usually involves surgery, chemotherapy and radiotherapy, or a combination of all three. Around 65% of people with bowel cancer will require surgery. In most cases surgery is a major procedure, often resulting in a stoma or colostomy bag. You may even have two or more major surgeries, and when combined with chemotherapy and radiotherapy, the whole treatment process can be long drawn out and challenging.

As an exercise professional, I'm deeply passionate about physical activity and the role it can play in recovery after illness and surgery. I've witnessed at first hand, time and time again, how rehabilitation and exercise therapy can completely change the course of recovery and long-term outcomes in people with bowel cancer, helping them to rebuild confidence and enabling them to lead a life of acceptance, movement and health, rather than one of fear and inactivity.

We all know that being active is good for our health. Moving more, sitting less and being physically active are known to reduce the risk of heart disease, stroke, diabetes, cancer and many other chronic conditions. But when it comes to bowel cancer, exercise could well be one of the most powerful tools in your armoury.

Experts in exercise oncology are calling for physical activity to be seen as the fourth treatment option for bowel cancer, and for it to be included as standard in the care package for anyone with the disease.[2]

And there is a growing body of scientific research to back up this bold claim. Being active will help you overcome many of the debilitating side-effects from chemotherapy and radiotherapy, such as fatigue, muscle loss and weakness. It can help your body tolerate the treatments better and there is emerging evidence that exercise may help your body fight the cancer cells. Some studies show that being active after a diagnosis of colorectal cancer can improve your chance of survival by around 20–30%.[3]

But above all, being active gives you a sense of wellbeing and control and boosts your psychological health. It helps you feel that you're doing something for yourself. And it just makes you feel better.

Yet I also know that exercise is one of the most difficult things to do when you have bowel cancer.

Despite the research, the messages from medical professionals about exercise are mixed and contradictory. There is very little practical encouragement to be active, and not much in the way of supervised exercise classes or groups. The 'rest is best' message is unfortunately very pervasive in society, so people aren't getting the encouragement they need. If the doctor says to rest, then that's what you'll do.

Some research (awaiting publication) I did in 2018 (on behalf of medical devices company ConvaTec.co.uk) found that 90% of people who had bowel cancer said they didn't do enough exercise for good health, as recommended by the World Health Organization (150 minutes of moderate activity per week).

To be fair, the vast majority of the population aren't active enough for good health, so it's no wonder when you have a cancer diagnosis it becomes even more difficult.

But it's still a terrifying statistic. If you're not meeting guidelines for exercise, you increase your risk of other co-morbidities – diabetes, heart disease, depression, arthritis etc – and fall into a vicious circle of inactivity and worsening quality of life. And we know that around 70% of people with cancer have at least one other chronic condition.

We need to reverse this trend. And fast! And that's the reason for this book.

Patients with bowel cancer need to get moving and feel confident around exercise; they need not to be scared of exercise or allow the barriers they face to prevent them being active.

But it's hard to know where to start, or what's safe. What sort of exercises should you do after surgery? Can you exercise with a stoma? How much exercise can you do when you're having chemo? What if you just don't feel like it? And how are you meant to get active when you feel exhausted and sick?

This book will help to answer all these questions and more.

It will help you navigate the confusing messages about exercise, how to overcome the barriers and how to feel more positive and motivated, even if you've never been active in the past.

You might be sceptical, uninterested or just too unwell to think about exercise. Don't dismiss it just yet. All I ask is you have a read of this book and give it a chance.

It may require a shift in your mindset but try to think about what you can do rather than what you can't.

Here's a 10-point guide to how this book can help people with bowel cancer:

Reason #1

First things first. It is completely safe to be active when you have bowel cancer. In fact, not only is it safe, but it should be viewed as part of your treatment and recovery plan. Some studies have shown that by being active after diagnosis, you can reduce the risk of recurrence of colon cancer by around 20–30%.[3] Chapter 1 shows that physical exercise can easily be built into your everyday life and does not have to include athletic or sporting activities if these are not your thing. You don't have to go to the gym to exercise. Being 'active' really means just sitting less and moving more. It doesn't have to be hard and it definitely does not have to hurt. Exercise needs to nourish you, not punish you.

Reason #2

Although you may not feel much like it, being active when you're having chemotherapy and radiotherapy can help to combat some of the side-effects and long-term consequences of treatment, such as muscle loss, weakness and fatigue. Chapter 2 describes the effects of different types of cancer treatment on the body and shows that even short 10-minute walks will make a huge difference. Little and often is best.

Reason #3

Even if you have advanced cancer, bone metastases or a complex condition, it's still okay for you to be active. As Chapter 3 shows, there may be some sensible adaptations you need to make, or you may need to work under the supervision of an exercise specialist or physio, but some sort of movement is one of the best things you can do to help you cope with cancer treatments and for quality of life.

Reason #4

After all abdominal surgery, and particularly if you have a stoma, you absolutely must do core/abdominal rehab exercises. Chapter 4 explains how to start them within a few days after your operation. It's essential to strengthen these muscles and restore the function of your core. Even though some doctors and nurses are cautious, clinical nursing guidelines[4] advise that it's safe to start 3–4 days after stoma surgery with appropriate exercises, and these are carefully explained to get you started.

Reason #5

It might seem counterintuitive, but exercise is a great way to overcome cancer-related/ chemotherapy fatigue. As Chapter 5 explains, studies show that doing some gentle exercise (short walks to start with) can actually help you feel more energised and reduce your feelings of fatigue. Try it and see how you feel.

Reason #6

The mental and psychological effects of exercise are immeasurable and incredibly powerful. Using movement as a way to recover after surgery and treatment will help you to rebuild your body, confidence, self-esteem and energy levels. In fact, I think the mental aspect of exercise is the most important of all, giving you a sense of control and positivity. Chapter 6 gives you an insight into how much exercise to do to facilitate your recovery, so that you don't over-do it and become demoralised, and lose out on the mental uplift exercise can give you.

Reason #7

Rest is not best for anyone, even when you have bowel cancer. By resting too much, you risk becoming even weaker and deconditioning even more… and falling into the inactivity/fear avoidance/loss of confidence spiral. Specifically, as Chapter 7 shows, after surgery you do not need to 'rest' for 6–12 weeks; instead, you should gradually start to become more active, walking more and beginning to do core exercises. Each exercise is carefully explained and illustrated to help you get started.

Reason #8

You can continue to exercise throughout treatment if you feel well enough. Chapter 8 gives a wide range of more advanced exercises you can try. You may need to adapt your training level or certain exercises for a while, but if you feel well there is no reason why you shouldn't increase your exercise routine if you want to. You just have to listen to your body.

Reason #9

Eating well and being active go hand in hand. To enable you to be physically active you need to nourish your body with the right food and fluids. After bowel surgery your diet may change, and you may feel you can't eat healthily or that your diet is restricted in some way. Chapter 9 covers the challenging topic of how to eat healthily after bowel surgery and offers some tips on making small changes to the food you eat to boost your recovery and long-term health.

Reason #10

Finally, Chapter 10 addresses the mind barriers that cancer patients often face when contemplating exercise. You don't have to feel 100% well to exercise. It's okay to start feeling tired or even quite unwell. Just moving a bit, going for a walk, doing some gentle stretches or something like yoga can actually help you feel better. You may have to push yourself to get started, but once you're going, you'll realise your body can do more than you thought.

But I also know it's not that easy.

The overall aim of this book is to provide a kind, gentle and understanding approach. To be empathic and encouraging, not judgemental. I simply want you to find out how exercise and proper nutrition can have a huge role in helping you feel better, rebuild your confidence and take control of your health, at a time when you feel most vulnerable.

There is a huge gap in patient care after bowel surgery. If you have a heart attack or have heart surgery, you usually get cardiac rehab. After a knee or hip replacement there's often physio and group rehab classes. And if you have a lung condition, you can benefit from pulmonary rehab exercise classes. But what if you have bowel cancer or a stoma? At the moment, there is very little support, knowledge or advice. I know that because as well as it being my own experience, I've surveyed thousands of patients with stomas and bowel cancer and the vast majority were never given any advice about exercise or rehabilitation. Too often people are told what they can't do, and there's very little support to tell them what they can do.

So, I hope this book goes some way to plugging that gap – providing you with some expert knowledge about safe exercise and specific core muscle rehabilitation, how to get moving again, how to eat well, and most importantly of all, how to rebuild your confidence.

You might also like to share the book with friends and family, so they can support and encourage you too.

Good luck. And remember…

When it comes to exercise, something is always possible, and something is always better than nothing.

Sarah Russell
2019
(Revised for reprint 2021)

PART I

KEEP MOVING, KEEP IMPROVING

Chapter 1

What do we mean by exercise?

Values and confidence scales

Before we go any further, I want you to explore your relationship with exercise and physical activity. How are you feeling reading this book about exercise and activity? Is it already making you feel overwhelmed or confused? Or is it beginning to help you feel more positive and confident?

Let's explore what exercise means to you, your relationship with exercise and how you feel about it.

You may be reading this having just come home from hospital, or during a particularly brutal bout of chemo, or you may be months down the line starting to recover. It doesn't matter where you are in relation to your treatment, I just want you to think about how you value and feel about exercise at this moment in time. We'll check back on this several times throughout the book to see whether your feelings change, and your confidence grows.

Score each question on the next page to reflect how you feel about physical activity at the moment.

- How important is it for you to be physically active right now?

1 Not at all important	2	3	4	5	6	7	8	9	10 Extremely important

- How confident do you feel about being physically active right now?

1 Not at all confident	2	3	4	5	6	7	8	9	10 Extremely confident

Let's 're-think' exercise

Changing our thoughts and feelings about 'exercise' might be the most important thing we can do to help get us moving more and have a happier relationship with physical activity. People say they're not 'sporty' or they don't like going to the gym, or that 'exercise' isn't for them. But physical activity shouldn't be something that's optional or only done when you have a bit of spare time. It needs to be integrated deeply into our lives and become part of our armoury against disease, mental illness, modern living and, in particular, against cancer. It deserves to be given the highest priority and should be seen as being as important as any medical treatment.

Everyone knows they should be more active. But the reality is that we are doing the opposite. We are living increasingly sedentary lives, and this is having a seriously negative effect on our health. This sedentary living is driving the increase in type 2 diabetes, heart disease, obesity, stroke, arthritis, dementia and even some cancers. It's a time bomb on a global scale.

If we don't get enough movement in our day-to-day lives – through our work, commute or home life – then we have to make a conscious choice to do something 'active' for our health, such as go for a walk, a run or to a class. And that is much harder to do. Humans are hard-wired to take the easiest option.

So how do we shift this mindset?

I've worked in the exercise industry for over 25 years. I've worked with thousands of clients over more than two decades and whilst I love everything to do with fitness, I think we need to fundamentally reframe our relationship with activity and exercise. It's become skewed by modern living, social media and technology. We need to step back and reassess why and how we do it and, more importantly, what it means to us.

What's the difference between exercise, physical activity and movement?

There is a subtle difference.

- 'Exercise' is defined as being purposeful and something that you might do with the aim of getting fit or improving your health. There is a clear goal and purposeful intention. Some examples might be going for a run or going to the gym.
- 'Physical activity' is defined as something that involves bodily movement *as a consequence rather than as a goal*. So, some good examples of this might be walking to work or doing some gardening or housework.
- 'Movement' is just that. Literally any kind of bodily movement involving the muscular skeletal system. This might simply be taking regular breaks from sitting at your computer or TV, or walking around your house, climbing stairs or just not being 'sedentary'.

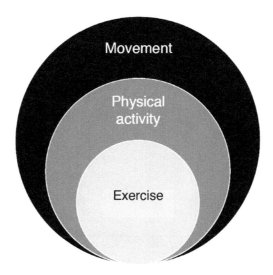

Figure 1.1 The relationship between exercise, physical activity and movement

As Figure 1.1 shows, all three are intertwined and equally important, but if you're feeling unwell or you've just had surgery, the thought of formal 'exercise' might be far from your mind for a while. But don't dismiss the benefits of 'movement' or just being 'active'. These form the foundation that comes before formal exercise and activity and may be more relevant depending on where you are in your recovery and treatment pathway.

Understanding the difference between exercise, physical activity and movement can be useful. It helps us break down barriers and understand our relationship with 'exercise'. When we talk about 'activity' or 'moving', it just seems less intimidating and more appealing. The word 'exercise' can be overwhelming. Exercise is often promoted as something that is hard work or involves going to the gym or getting up a sweat. And I think it's why it can be off-putting for so many. But as you'll find out later, it really doesn't need to be. A gentler approach to exercise has many more benefits.

What 'exercise' means to me

I do the following activity with groups of nurses during training courses. I ask them to draw a picture or write some words to describe whatever comes into their head when they think of the word 'exercise'. I want you to do the same in the box below.

> What comes into my head when I hear the word 'exercise':

Almost all the nurses draw people swimming, running, playing football, going to the gym or some other formal exercise or sport, or write words such as 'tiring', 'pain', 'hard work', 'sweaty!'. What did you draw or write? Did you do the same as the nurses?

But as explained earlier there are many other forms of movement and activity which are just as relevant and beneficial for our health.

Think of simple daily activities such as walking, housework, gardening, DIY or washing the car, for example. These activities have huge benefits for your health and count as physical activity (if you get a bit out of breath doing them), but hardly anyone would choose to write them down as a form of 'exercise'.

But why not? I think that's where we're going wrong. We've developed an 'all or nothing' approach to exercise which does nothing for our engagement with long-term movement.

Your exercise relationship

Next, I want you to write down a bit about your previous relationship with exercise, prior to your diagnosis. In the box provided below, answer the following questions:
- What physical activities did I enjoy before cancer? (Everything counts… DIY, housework, dog walking, dancing, gym, running, cycling etc.)
- What did I enjoy about these activities? How did they make me feel? What did I get out of it? How did my body feel?

The physical activities I enjoyed before cancer were:

They made me feel:

And now let's look at what's changed since your diagnosis. Score your answers to the questions on the next page on the scales provided.

- How active am I right now?

1 Very sedentary	2	3	4	5	6	7	8	9	10 Extremely active

- How satisfied do I feel about my activity level at present?

1 Very unhappy	2	3	4	5	6	7	8	9	10 Extremely satisfied

And finally, answer the following questions in the box provided.
- What's changed?
- How do I feel about exercise now?
- Are there things I feel I can't do that I did before?
- Why is that? What are the things that make it difficult?

Just going through this task and writing things down may have triggered some thoughts or feelings you didn't know you had, so come back to it later if you found it difficult.

So where are we going wrong with 'exercise'?

A quick Google search for the word 'exercise' brings up images of muscular bodies in tight Lycra and people running, doing weights or at the gym. There are messages about 'no excuses', 'no pain no gain' and 'not quitting'. Most are doing exercises designed to 'tone' an area of their body or lose weight and it just feels intimidating and hard. There is very little about health and mental wellbeing and none of it feels 'nourishing' and gentle.

This sends the message that how we look and what we weigh are the most important things and that unless we're 'smashing it' in the gym, it's not worth doing. I think these messages can be really damaging and lead people to think about exercise in 'black and white' terms. And it's not helpful when we need to think about exercise and physical activity in the context of cancer.

Instead, let's think about the 'health' benefits of being active, rather than how we look. We need to focus on having strong muscles and a strong body and on being able to walk, run, lift things and be active for our health.

We need to think of 'movement' as a way to prevent disease, treat conditions and help us FEEL good, rather than just to lose weight or tone up. A bit like another type of medication or nourishing food. It needs to become part of life. A habit as ingrained as brushing your teeth.

Intuitive movement

Instead of exercise being an activity which requires hard work and pain, exercise can become something gentler, more intuitive – yet still with huge benefits. It can become a lifestyle choice to *move more*, integrated into everyday life so that it becomes a 'way of being' and a way of life.

If your brain associates exercise with pain, you'll eventually stop doing it. So, I tend to encourage people to exercise more gently, not to constantly push themselves. I believe that this helps people to develop a healthy relationship with activity and learn to love it… and more importantly, to keep doing it for the rest of their lives. I'd rather see longevity than fast results.

What is 'intuitive movement'?

Intuitive exercise/movement doesn't have an official definition. It's more of an ethos.

I'd describe it as an approach to exercise where you feel at peace with your relationship with your body, how it looks, how it feels and how it works. It's a sense of knowing what your body needs. When to move, when to rest. Being *really* tuned in to how your muscles and mind feel, and what they need to be healthy.

It's probably the opposite of the current fitness culture. It's about finding a way to be active that you love. That makes you feel great both during and afterwards. It doesn't injure you or hurt you and it's not competitive, but it pushes you just enough to see health results. Being intuitive with exercise is NOT about 'numbers', weight loss, burning calories, setting goals, beating yourself up or feeling guilty. It's about being active for health, for mental wellbeing and for lifelong enjoyment.

It took for me to go through illness and life-changing surgery to really 'get it'. But now I do, I want to share it with everyone I meet, coach and work with. And this approach is especially important when you have cancer or any other illness.

How to become more intuitive with exercise

The following tips are just to get you thinking about your approach to activity in general.

1. Change the way you think about 'exercise'... call it 'movement' or 'activity' if you prefer. Move away from the 'all or nothing' approach. Ten minutes' brisk walking is great and can bring many health benefits. You don't have to go to the gym or a formal class or group. If you want to, that's great, but there are a million and one other ways to be active.

2. Find ways to incorporate more movement into your everyday life. Find opportunities to move, rather than to take the easy option. Wash your own car rather than using the carwash, take the stairs rather than a lift, use a push mower rather than a ride-on, walk to work or to the shops instead of taking the car, use a standing desk, do some stretching whilst watching TV. All of this will get you into a 'movement' frame of mind, rather than a sedentary one.

3. Harder is not better. Exercise does not have to be hard to be effective. Gentle movement has huge health benefits. Try to put in enough effort so that you're breathing a little harder and your heartrate increases, but you can still chat. If you can't chat, then you're exercising too hard. Of course, there is a place for higher intensity exercise too but if you're exercising 'intuitively' you'll feel

when you want to push harder and when your body is ready for it.

4. Focus on exercise for 'health' rather than for how you look or what you weigh (in fact, throw out the scales). Dissociate exercise from body image and weight. Instead I want you to concentrate on health outcomes and mental wellbeing. How does being active make you feel? Do you sleep better? Can you feel your stress levels reducing? Do you feel less anxious? In time are you noticing stronger muscles in your legs? Are you able to go a little further or a little faster with your walk or run? How about your relationships? Can you spend time with your family doing activity or make new friends?

5. Ditch the fitness apps and online challenges which offer instant fitness or fast results, especially the '30-day challenge' ones. There are no quick fixes. Think about movement and exercise as a lifelong relationship. It may ebb and flow throughout your life and have a different meaning at various stages, but it will always be there for you as a close friend.

6. When exercising and moving, think about how you feel and the level of effort in your body. Listen to your body DURING and AFTER exercise or activity. Is your heart beating faster? Is your breathing rate going up? Are you sweating? Are your muscles working? Which muscles can you feel working? Do you have any aches or pains or areas of tightness?

7. Be mindful. Be aware of your surroundings. If you're outdoors, what can you see? Notice the weather, the warmth of the sun or the wind on your skin. Notice the crunch of leaves under your feet. The birds in the sky. Notice the sun and the clouds. Feel the rain on your face. Breathe in the fresh air.

8. Be aware of social connection and friendships. This is one of the most underestimated aspects of activity and exercise. It might be more effort to go out to meet a friend or go to a class, but the social connections and support you'll receive will have a huge impact on your health and wellbeing. Who are you with? Are you laughing and having fun? Enjoy having a shared experience with a friend or family member. You're creating lifelong memories.

9. Be patient. Allow your 'fitness' to come to you, rather than chasing it too hard. Avoid setting specific targets or goals. Instead, focus on daily behaviours, mindset and tuning in to your body's needs. The rest will take care of itself.

You might be wondering what this has to do with your cancer. I'm pretty sure that this approach to exercise is the key to overcoming many of the barriers we have around exercise and health. And when you're dealing with cancer, you need to break down as many barriers as possible and find a way to incorporate exercise into your life in a different way.

Reset your relationship with exercise and how you feel about movement, and you're halfway there.

And finally, let's just revisit those scales from the beginning of the chapter.

- How important is it for you to be physically active right now?

1 Not at all important	2	3	4	5	6	7	8	9	10 Extremely important

- How confident do you feel about being physically active right now?

1 Not at all confident	2	3	4	5	6	7	8	9	10 Extremely confident

Compare your scores here with your scores from the beginning of this chapter. I hope that they have gone up and you're feeling more positive just by reading this chapter.

Key points

- If you were active before your cancer diagnosis, everything can change. You can lose your confidence and lose trust in your body. You don't know where to start, your body feels different and you can't do the things you used to. This can make it difficult to re-engage with the activities you did before.
- Even if you know you should be active, it's incredibly hard and there are multiple barriers. Knowing and doing are two very different things. You know you *should* but somehow, it's too difficult. This can make you feel even

worse, especially if you try and can't manage it. That does nothing to build confidence and it's easy to spiral into negativity and declining motivation.

• We need to find ways to make exercise and activity more achievable, enjoyable and doable. We need to 're-frame' the concept of exercise and soften it. In a nutshell, we need to make it something we associate with pleasant thoughts and responses rather than dreading it. Exercise should be nourishing, not punishing.

• And THAT is the bit that's so important for people with cancer, regardless of whether you're going through treatment or are on the road to recovery. Feeling vulnerable and unwell makes it even harder to exercise and be active. You need as much knowledge, information, support and encouragement as possible to help you overcome the barriers and get moving.

• The irony is that if you can overcome some of these barriers, being active can be the very thing to help you feel better, physically and emotionally. You'll develop your confidence again and you can enjoy the wonderful health benefits that exercise and movement have to offer. It may not be easy, but with some simple tweaks and a mindset shift, you can find a way.

Chapter 2

Treatments for bowel cancer and how exercise can help

Now let's look at how cancer treatment affects your body and your ability to be active. Generally speaking, there are three main types of treatment for bowel cancer: surgery, chemotherapy and radiotherapy. Other targeted, biological and immunotherapy treatments are also available for some patients, although less common.

Some people will have a combination of all treatments, including surgery, some may just have surgery without chemotherapy or radiotherapy. It depends on the location and stage of your cancer, as well as decisions made by your oncology team and your own personal choices.

Here are some of the most common treatments and a simple explanation of how they work, affect your body and how exercise can help specifically.

Chemotherapy

Chemotherapy works by stopping the growth of cancer cells – which are growing and dividing rapidly – in your body. Chemotherapy also kills any other *growing* cells in your body, including your hair, skin, bone marrow and lining of your mouth and intestines. This is why you can lose your hair, have impaired immunity and often suffer from gastrointestinal issues during chemotherapy.

There are many different types of chemotherapy and ways of receiving the treatment and everyone is different in terms of how they respond and the side-effects they have. Some people have a lot of side-effects and others have none.

The main side-effects that people report are fatigue, anaemia, impaired immunity and nausea, but there can also be longer-term effects of chemotherapy, including other cancers, heart and lung changes, muscle loss and bone weakness, arthritis, neurological changes and weight gain.

It not a list that makes for happy reading, but the positive news is that many of these consequences can be offset and improved with physical activity and exercise. In particular fatigue, muscle loss and bone weakness.

Radiotherapy

Radiotherapy involves the use of high-energy X-ray beams to treat the tumour and destroy the cancer cells. It's generally given by an external X-ray beam over a period of weeks. The radiotherapy beam can also do damage to other normal cells in the surrounding tissue, organs and skin. These cells can repair over time, unlike cancer cells which are permanently destroyed.

The main side-effect of radiotherapy is cumulative fatigue, which builds up as the treatment goes on. Sometimes this is at its worst when treatment is over. Other consequences can include bone weakness, lymphoedema and gastrointestinal issues. As with chemotherapy, it's likely that most symptoms – fatigue in particular – can be helped by appropriate activity.

Surgery

The majority of people with colorectal cancer will have surgery to remove the tumour and a section of bowel. It's common to be given a stoma (often referred to as a colostomy bag) – where you wear a bag on your abdomen to collect your waste instead of going to the toilet in the normal way. This is done to divert the bowel during treatment, to allow the bowel to heal after surgery and sometimes is temporary and reversed at a later date (but not always). Some surgeries are done using the 'keyhole' method (laparoscopic surgery) where small incisions are made; other surgery is performed by making a large wound vertically (laparotomy) up your abdomen. This will depend on your surgeon and location of the tumour.

In some people, where the cancer has spread to surrounding tissue or other organs, they may need extensive surgery to remove pelvic organs and pelvic muscles, and reconstructive surgery is sometimes needed. Pelvic exenteration is an operation where multiple pelvic organs are removed – bowel, bladder and female reproductive organs. It's major surgery and you may need a colostomy and/or a urostomy, along with reconstructive surgery for the pelvic floor or vagina.

The main issue with any abdominal surgery is tissue/muscle damage and pain around the surgical area. As the surgeon has to cut through muscle in your abdomen, there will also be weakness and reduced function in your core muscles. Full 'healing' of the wounds usually takes around 6–12 weeks, again depending on the type of surgery, and everyone is different.

This is where exercise and early rehabilitation have a huge part to play. Damaged tissue goes through phases of repair as it starts to heal. Movement and gentle exercise during these early phases can improve the healing process – increasing blood flow, reducing scar tissue and improving range of movement and muscle strength.

Talk to your surgeon, physiotherapist or nurse first, but you should aim to start gentle movement and rehabilitation exercises within days after surgery. This will help to speed up your recovery and will rebuild your confidence – so try not to be too cautious and fearful.

Pre-habilitation – preparing for bowel cancer surgery

If you were going to run a marathon you would prepare your body and get as fit as possible. The marathon places huge strain on your body and to run it without training would be difficult. If you weren't fit enough, you might have to drop out half way or you might become ill or injured. Your performance might not be very good, your recovery afterwards would take much longer, your muscles would be sore and you'd be more likely to get an injury and have complications.

Preparing for bowel surgery is very similar to running a marathon. Much like marathon running, bowel surgery places considerable strain on your body and the fitter you are going into it, the better your recovery and outcomes from surgery. The term 'pre-habilitation' is used to describe the process of getting fit BEFORE bowel cancer surgery. It's becoming a big area of research and many trials are being run around the world looking at different interventions, some at hospitals in the UK. Studies so far are showing that people who are frail going into surgery often don't do as well, so getting fitter before their operation can mean reduced risk of complications and better recovery. As little as four weeks of exercise in the 'pre-surgery' phase is enough to improve physical fitness and make a difference to outcomes – less readmission, better long-term outcomes, fewer complications and, in some cases, lower mortality. If you're reading this BEFORE your operation, then speak to your surgeon/oncologist about whether a pre-habilitation programme is something that can be offered to you.

If it's not, then you'll have to plan your own approach and put an exercise programme into action yourself. Harder to do, but not impossible. Even if you just have a few weeks before your operation, there's still plenty you can do.

How much you can do will depend on your current fitness level and health condition. Little and often is best. Use the guidelines in Chapters 6, 7 and 8 to help structure what you do – monitoring your heartrate and intensity levels.

Waiting for surgery can be stressful. But people say that having something practical and positive to focus on really helps them cope.

Targeted, biological and immunotherapies

New cancer treatments are being developed all the time; targeted, biological and immunotherapies are seen as new and hopeful ways to treat specific cancers, although not suitable for everyone and, in some cases, they are still in trial phases. These treatments are all very different, but generally work by trying to target the way in which the cancer cells grow and replicate. Immunotherapy works by unleashing your own immune system on the cancer cells. Side-effects vary from person to person and treatment type, but can include flu symptoms, fatigue and pain/soreness at the needle site. Because there are so many different types of treatment it's impossible to say how you will be affected. Speak to your nurse or oncologist about your individual treatment and side-effects that you might expect.

The mental and physical impact of bowel cancer

The mental and physical consequences of any treatment are often the most troubling aspect of bowel cancer and can be tough to cope with. In many cases, you may not have had any symptoms of bowel cancer; your cancer was picked up by screening and now suddenly you're having surgery and chemo and are feeling worse than you did before. It can be a huge shock and a very scary time.

If you've had more than one type of treatment – and many people do – you could well be struggling with a whole range of debilitating side-effects. And that can make it hard just to get out of bed, let alone think about exercise or being active.

And this is where you need to rethink everything you know about exercise and shift your mindset about the traditional sedentary 'recovery' as often prescribed.

A common response is to wait until it's all over, put life on hold until treatment has ended and then to think about being active again. Try to resist this and, although it won't be easy, try to find ways to be active *during* your treatment. Putting life on hold could mean being inactive for months, if not a year or more. You'll feel so much better, cope with the side-effects better and speed up your recovery (and potentially improve survival) if you can integrate some activity into your treatment pathway.

 · Think about physical activity as another type of treatment. One that is equally as important as your chemo, radiotherapy or surgery. One that can be used alongside any of these treatments to offset some of those side-effects, aid your recovery and improve your long-term outcome. It's like having another medicine available to you.

However, it's probably no surprise to learn that research by the Macmillan Cancer Charity[1] found that many people with bowel cancer become less active after their diagnosis. This can then last for many years, with some people never regaining the same level of activity again, even when fully recovered. Maybe you feel like this yourself?

The shock of the diagnosis, treatment side-effects and physical changes, combined with loss of confidence and fear, can leave people in a vicious circle of negativity. This can lead to ongoing inactivity, poor quality of life and a sense of not living life to the fullest (see Figure 2.1).

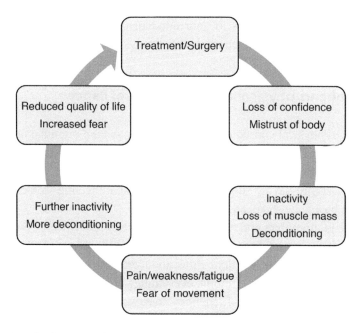

Figure 2.1 The fear–avoidance – inactivity – reduced quality of life vicious circle

Without some kind of intervention – an exercise group, rehab class or similar – you can end up staying in this cycle. It can be very hard to become active again or start to exercise for the first time. And this cycle can go on and on, unless an intervention is put in place to break the chain.

In an ideal world, that 'intervention' needs to be a programme of physical activity, ideally some sort of rehabilitation or cancer-appropriate fitness group or class, led by a qualified exercise professional or oncology physiotherapist. There are examples all over the world which include dance classes, football clubs, walking groups and specific circuit exercise groups, all of which have huge benefits for the people who attend.

It doesn't have to be a cancer-specific rehab group – these sorts of groups are like gold dust, so if you have one locally that you can attend, then you're lucky. Any kind of appropriate exercise group would be suitable. One with a qualified cancer rehabilitation instructor is ideal, but, if not, you can monitor your own exercise intensity and modify any exercises as required.

Most people just need a little reassurance and encouragement that it's safe to exercise and some guidelines and structure to approach it. And hopefully that's what this book will do.

You're going to have to think about all the ways in which you can be active and develop your own intervention. What do you enjoy doing? How can family and friends help? What facilities or local classes have you got? What can you do at home? Would the neighbour's dog like to go for a walk?

What's the relationship between exercise and bowel cancer?

The world of exercise oncology (the study of the relationship between cancer and exercise) is moving at a rapid pace and it's an exciting time. Over the last few years, the evidence has become much stronger that not only is exercise safe for cancer patients, but that it has an important place in the treatment and management of cancer.

The evidence is now so strong, that, as mentioned in the Introduction, in 2018 the Clinical Oncology Society Australia (COSA) published a position statement[2] calling for exercise to be a standard part of care for ALL cancer patients. This means that everyone with cancer should be supported to be active, to attend an exercise class/group of some sort and for it to be integrated alongside chemotherapy, surgery, radiotherapy and other treatments.

The research is ongoing, but there seem to be a number of specific biological mechanisms which explain how exercise helps during and after cancer.

1. Exercise lowers levels of hormones in the body, in particular insulin and oestrogen and certain growth factors, which are associated with cancer development and disease progression.
2. Being active is associated with reducing obesity and decreasing the effects of being overweight – especially the development of insulin resistance. There is a strong link between type 2 diabetes and cancer for this reason.
3. Regular exercise (along with a healthy diet, healthy gut microbiome and plenty of sleep) reduces inflammation in the body – chronic low-grade inflammation is associated with a number of chronic diseases as well as cancer.
4. Moderate-intensity exercise boosts the immune function – meaning that you may be able to tolerate your treatment better and have more consistent treatment which will be more effective.
5. Exercise speeds up your digestive system and reduces the amount of time it takes for food to travel through the intestines (transit time). This reduces exposure time to possible carcinogens (substances which are known to cause cancer), especially in the colon/large intestines, and thereby reduces the risk of bowel cancer developing. And more importantly for you, some studies have shown that being active AFTER a diagnosis of bowel cancer can reduce the risk of recurrence by up to 20–30%.[3]
6. And finally, there are some early studies that show exercise may in fact help some treatments work better and aid your body in fighting the cancer cells.

Reducing side-effects

The side-effects of treatment and surgery can be the hardest thing to cope with. It seems counterintuitive, but being active during and after treatment is one of the best ways to combat some of those debilitating consequences.

As explained in Chapter 1, you don't need to feel 'totally well' in order to exercise. We have this misconception that before you can be active, you need to be feeling 100%. It's simply not true. Even if you're feeling quite unwell, if you can just get moving a bit, go for a walk, do some exercises at home or even just some gentle stretching, the chances are you'll feel better as a RESULT of doing some exercise.

Being active can:
- reduce fatigue
- help you sleep better and combat insomnia
- improve heart health
- prevent muscle loss
- manage your weight – gain or loss
- prevent bone loss and improve bone strength
- improve appetite
- prevent constipation
- improve mental wellbeing and boost confidence.

Let's look at some of these benefits in more detail.

Fatigue

Chapter 5 covers this in more detail, but fatigue is the most common and debilitating side-effect reported by almost all cancer patients, affecting 70–80% of people.[4] Multiple studies have shown that being active is one of the best ways to combat fatigue.[5] Although it's not known exactly how, gentle aerobic exercise seems to be the best and could even prevent fatigue taking hold in the first place. One likely explanation is the increase in red blood cells in people who are active, compared with those who are sedentary. It also boosts endorphins and other hormones – and just gets you feeling more energised.

Muscle strength

All cancer treatments can cause muscle loss. This is a direct effect of the cancer and treatment combined with moving less, periods of being in bed or hospital and changes in nutrition. It's well established that 10 days in a hospital bed can result in 10% muscle loss or the equivalent of ageing 10 years.[6,7] It's that feeling of being 'weak as a kitten' after surgery or treatment. You feel like you've lost all muscle, and normal day-to-day activities can feel really difficult. That might sound very familiar to you?

Muscle loss then results in loss of balance, increased risk of falls, general weakness and a sense of vulnerability. In my mind it's probably the most significant problem affecting almost all cancer patients. And unfortunately, continued rest will make muscle loss worse. It's a vicious circle. Chapter 6 explains how to break the cycle.

Bone strength

Reduction in bone strength is another common effect of treatment. Treatments (chemotherapy, radiotherapy) can lead to thinning of the bone – known as osteoporosis – which can increase your risk of fractures for many months and years to come.

Bone strength is directly linked to muscle strength too. If you're inactive and lose muscle, then you're likely to suffer bone weakness as well. Exercise – in particular resistance activity – can prevent or even reverse bone weakness.

See Chapter 3 for detailed advice on what to do if you have, or are at high risk of, osteosporosis.

Can exercise reduce recurrence of cancer?

Recurrence is one of the biggest worries for anyone with bowel cancer. However, the good news is that it may be possible to reduce your risk of recurrence by around 30% by being active and doing some exercise after your diagnosis and treatment.[8]

The evidence in this area is growing fast and becoming more and more compelling.[5] Colorectal cancer and the link with exercise is widely researched, and it seems that exercise has the biggest effect in terms of prevention and recurrence, compared with others such as breast, prostate or lung. It's thought this is primarily due to the mechanism of improving transit time through the gut. Even though it's early days for the evidence, I can't think of a better motivator to be active.

Whilst there isn't an agreement about exactly HOW MUCH exercise you need to do to reduce your risk just yet, most of the studies are based on a minimum of meeting the physical activity guidelines of 150 minutes per week. So as a minimum, try to do 20 minutes of something every day, or 30 minutes on five days of the week.

But there seems to be a dose response. The more you can do, the lower your risk. But anything is better than nothing, so just get moving and don't worry about how much you do.

The message is clear. Do as much as you can and lower your risk of your cancer coming back, along with other chronic conditions such as diabetes, heart disease and stroke.

Key points

- You don't have to feel 'well' in order to be active. The act of doing something active could actually be the thing that helps you feel better and gives you more energy.
- You don't have to 'love' exercise at the time… but do think about its effects afterwards. What it gives you, how it makes you feel and what you get out of it.
- Try not to put life on hold until treatment is over. It might last many months, if not years. Instead try to be active *during* treatment; in the gaps between surgeries or rounds of chemo. Think about physical activity as another form of therapy or treatment.
- Exercise is one of the best ways to combat many of the side-effects of cancer treatment, particularly fatigue. Little and often is best. Even 10-minute walks around the block will make a huge difference.
- Bone weakness and muscle loss are both commonly reported side-effects, leaving you feeling weak and vulnerable. Home-based resistance exercises can help to reduce treatment-related muscle loss and are simple and easy to do.
- Make a list of all the ways being active can help you. How does it make you feel afterwards? Almost everyone says they just 'feel better' for some movement and activity or that it helps them feel they are doing something positive. Write your own list about what you get out of exercise.
- Getting exercise intensity right can be tricky. You need to do it briskly enough to get benefits, but not too much that you end up exhausted and feeling worse. Use the intensity guidelines in Chapter 6 to guide you.
- Knowing the reasons why it's important to be active is unlikely to be enough to motivate you when you feel awful/tired/sick… so you'll need to dig deep and find strategies and friends to help you. You'll probably need to push yourself to get going, but once you do, you're likely to feel so much better.

PART II

STAYING SAFE

Chapter 3

Precautions and adaptations

This chapter provides some basic guidelines, precautions and safety considerations regarding exercise both during and after cancer treatment. In particular, it addresses issues such as whether you can exercise if you have had abdominal surgery, or have concerns about things like lymphoedema, PICC/port lines, peripheral neuropathy, bone metastases and other complications.

In addition to the guidelines here, do your own research, talk to your doctor, talk to other patients, and listen to your own body and make your own decisions about what is right for you. Every situation is different clinically and your decisions about what you do, the pros and cons, and how you live your life are very personal to you.

However, bear in mind that when it comes to exercise and cancer there are very few strict limitations and restrictions, and people often find they can do much more than they think. You may need to make some adaptations to certain movements, intensity, duration and weight, but the benefits of being active almost always outweigh any possible risks or harm.

In general:
- you CAN be active when you're having chemotherapy
- you CAN be active when you have a stoma (more in Chapter 4)
- you CAN be active when you are having radiotherapy
- you CAN get back to normal activities after bowel surgery, and
- you CAN use exercise to help you recover sooner.

Is it safe to exercise?

When it comes to exercising safely, there are some basic guidelines regarding more complex situations, side-effects and symptoms. For instance, I'd recommend you get a copy of *Physical Activity and Cancer*[1] published by Macmillan Cancer Support. But there are very few situations where it's advisable not to 'be active' at all, and for the most part your body will guide you. Use heartrate to monitor intensity (see Chapter 6), and fatigue scales to provide some feedback and guidance (see Chapter 5).

It can be hard to untangle your symptoms and treatment side-effects. Generally speaking, gentle movement and physical activity are rarely contra-indicated, even if you have complex symptoms and multiple conditions.

If you are feeling daunted, do remember the difference between 'exercise', 'movement' and 'physical activity' explained in Chapter 1. Moving a bit more, going for a walk or doing some mobility exercises at home, is very different from doing harder, more intense exercise (running or cycling, for example) where you might raise your heartrate and get out of breath.

There are hardly any situations where this sort of gentle exercise will do you harm. There may, however, be times when you need to adapt or modify high-intensity exercise, training volumes and expectations, especially if you were very active prior to diagnosis.

When we're thinking about 'whether it's safe to exercise', try not to think in black and white terms. There's a grey area where moving about a bit more, walking and home-based activities are generally appropriate for most people, even those who are very unwell or with advanced disease.

However, there are some general safety considerations to be aware of.

Consult your doctor BEFORE formal exercise if you have:
- low blood count/impaired immunity
- new/unusual chest, jaw or arm pain
- vomiting/diarrhoea
- fever or (whole body) systemic infection
- unusual/sudden muscular weakness
- irregular or unusually low or high heartrate
- recent fainting or dizziness
- bleeding from any source, especially new or unusual.

Reduce the intensity/volume or type of exercise and consult your doctor if you have:
- a severe skin reaction to radiotherapy
- recent bone, back or neck pain
- persistent, new or unusual headaches
- recent joint pain or swelling of a joint or limb.

Common FAQs

Can I do any activities involving lifting after abdominal surgery?

You'll most likely be advised to 'avoid heavy lifting' after surgery. Some clinicians advise lifting 'nothing more than a kettle' for six weeks. However, whilst it's important not to place strain on your abdominal wounds, this blanket 'ban' on lifting can be limiting and disabling and create more fear. What if you have a small child who wants a cuddle? Or what if you live alone and need to cook for yourself? 'Not lifting' anything at all isn't terribly practical, or necessary.

Instead I want you to think about lifting safely. HOW you lift something is far more important than WHAT you lift. Awkward lifting and moving can cause more strain than lifting a heavier load if you lift it well. How you use your body to lift, how well your core is working and how you position yourself in relation to the item you're lifting are all far more important considerations.

Lifting can be done in many different ways and you can reduce the strain on your core by lifting using the correct techniques. Let's say you want to lift a kettle to make a cup of tea. Think about how you do that activity without placing undue strain on your abdomen. Break it down into steps and try the following tips:
- Hold the kettle as close to your body (and the front of the countertop) as possible, using your arms to do the work.
- Only put a small amount of water into the kettle – only what you need for one cup of tea, for example.
- Tighten up your abdomen and pelvic floor muscles before you lift – just to create a bit of support and stability. See more about how to do this in Chapter 7.
- Use your opposite hand to brace (on the kitchen worktop) and provide support.
- Breathe out as you lift – exhale on the lifting part of the movement.

Get a feel for this technique and you can apply it to the way you lift anything.

Always 'breathe out' (or exhale) as you lift something. This reduces strain on your abdomen. Keep items that you want to lift close to your body and get your arms and legs to do the work.

Research has shown that getting up from a chair in the wrong way (holding your breath and bracing, pushing with your arms) can place more strain on your abdomen than lifting a 9 kilo (20 lb) weight from a counter top. This is to do with a concept known as 'intra-abdominal pressure' (IAP) and it's something to be aware of after surgery, especially if you have a stoma. See more about this in Chapter 4.

So, although I'm not suggesting you go out and lay a patio or carry heavy loads of laundry in the first few weeks after surgery, you are safe to lift smaller items and start to gradually introduce day-to-day activities such as carrying small bags of shopping, remembering the tips above.

The more you can strengthen your core muscles (see Chapter 7), the stronger you'll feel, and you'll be able to lift more safely and effectively.

I'm anaemic; can I exercise?

Anaemia is common in people with cancer, especially if you're having chemotherapy. It's a condition where your body doesn't have enough red blood cells. Red blood cells carry oxygen to the tissues in your body, so it can make you feel tired, breathless and light-headed and give you headaches. It's thought that almost all cancer patients having chemotherapy will be mildly anaemic, and many will have more severe anaemia. Your doctor will monitor you with regular blood tests and treat you if you develop anaemia.

Much will depend on how well you feel and how severe your anaemia is. Exercise has actually been shown to improve anaemia as regular aerobic exercise boosts red blood cells, but like everything, you need to get the balance right. If your anaemia is mild/moderate, then you should be safe to exercise at a low/moderate intensity (5–6 on the scale of intensity, or around 70–75% maximum heartrate – see Chapter 6). Brisk walking for 20–30 minutes per day is ideal.

See how you feel and adjust the intensity/duration accordingly. If a small amount of exercise makes you feel worse, then reduce the volume or intensity next time. If you feel okay, then monitor your recovery and gradually increase your exercise over time. If your anaemia, and symptoms, are more severe then speak with your doctor about whether it's okay for you to exercise. If you're severely anaemic, it's unlikely you'll feel up to doing much until it's been treated.

I have impaired immunity (immunosuppression); is it okay for me to exercise?

Cancer treatments can compromise your white blood cell count, and this can impair your immune system, making it more likely for you to pick up infections. When your white blood cell count is low (your doctor will monitor your blood and will let you know if there is a problem), you are at increased risk of infection. You can still exercise gently (light activity and movement) and it's important to do so, but avoid ill people, public places, gyms and swimming pools, and high-intensity exercise.

Limit contact with other people and make sure you only use clean equipment. Home exercise videos can be useful, or just go out walking or gentle jogging with a (healthy) friend and limit physical contact with people outside of your home.

This can pose a challenge, especially if you're used to going to the gym, pool or a fitness class, and it can cut you off from your exercise buddies. Dig into your 'growth mindset' (see page 64) and find alternatives for the short term until your immune system is back on track. And remember it's not a permanent state.

I have lymphoedema; what exercise is safe and what should I avoid?

Lymphoedema is a swelling of a limb and, although rare in colorectal cancer patients, it can occur in one or both legs. It is caused by a build-up of lymph, due to a disruption in the lymphatic system. It can occur if you've had lymph nodes removed or radiotherapy.

In general, exercise helps to pump lymph around the body, so it's important to keep moving and exercising in the right way, even if you have already developed lymphoedema. Some research has shown that starting an exercise programme soon after surgery may reduce the risk of lymphoedema developing, and regular exercise can reduce symptoms if you already have it.

Here's a list of things to consider.
- Any sort of gentle movement – things like swinging your limbs and pumping your ankles – will help to get the lymph moving and to reduce some of the symptoms.
- If your leg(s) are affected, keep them moving and try not to protect or immobilise them.
- Walking, cycling and daily activities are ideal to keep you moving.
- Swimming and being in water are an excellent form of exercise for anyone

with lymphoedema. The water pressure helps to 'massage' the lymphatic system and can reduce pressure and swelling.

- Build up resistance exercises in small and gradual increments. Mini squats or 'chair squats' are ideal.
- Wear a compression sleeve on your leg if it's prescribed by your nurse or care team.
- Your limbs may be more at risk of infection, so be careful if you're out in the woods or gardening in case you scratch your skin on a bramble or thorn.

For those who are very active

There are some considerations to bear in mind if you want to be more active/return to the gym etc.

- The ASCM (American College of Sports Medicine) recommends avoiding any static (isometric) exercises relating to the limb with lymphoedema. This is where you hold a position without moving – such as doing a wall sit, plank, box position (on hands and knees) or hold a heavy weight in the same position without moving it.
- Anything where you get a build-up of pressure in the limb, put a lot of force through it or get a feeling of increasing tightness, should probably be avoided.
- And whilst light weight training is fine, the ASCM also advises against extremely strenuous repetitive activities – lifting very heavy weights or multiple repetitions of the same movement (heavy weighted squats, leg press etc.).
- If you have lymphoedema in your leg, you'd be best to do squats or lunges instead, where you're moving through the exercise, rather than holding a static position.

Everyone is affected differently, and all you can do is monitor your limb(s) and watch for any changes. Speak to your nurse or oncology team if you're concerned.

Can I exercise safely with bone metastases/osteoporosis?

Yes, you can, just with some modifications.

People with diagnosed metastatic bone disease – where the cancer has spread to their bones – or those with osteoporosis/bone weakness or myeloma, are at increased risk of fracture. However, this doesn't mean not to exercise or avoid physical activity altogether. In fact, quite the opposite. It's important to keep the muscles and bones strong, so don't avoid activity.

It may just mean making some adjustments to any exercise programme or ways in which you move. Macmillan Cancer Care published a specific leaflet in 2018 on the subject entitled *Physical Activity for People with Metastatic Bone Disease*[2] to provide some guidelines and recommendations for exercise professionals. This is available online at the Macmillan website (see page 195).

A summary of these guidelines is as follows:

1. Exercise should be low impact (no jumping, hopping, running, landing etc) and a mixture of aerobic training and resistance training (weight bearing and non-weight bearing).
2. No exercise should cause pain over the area of the metastases.
3. Any new symptoms must be investigated before continuing to exercise.
4. Avoid exercises that would result in quick rotation of your torso or shear forces over areas of known bone fragility, so avoid rapid twists and rotations, especially with load/weight.

The message is very clear, that physical activity has many benefits for people with bone metastases/fracture risk. People should try to be as active as possible within their capabilities. It's important to keep your bones and muscles as strong as possible; this will reduce the risk of falls, and potentially the risk of a fracture occurring.

Here are some things to consider.

- Resistance exercises at home or in a gym setting, using weights, a stretchy band (theraband) or body weight are good – where you do a number of repetitions of the same exercise.
- Exercises such as bicep curls, squats, sit-stands, lunges or seated exercises using a stretchy band (theraband) – are all ideal. Try 8–12 repetitions and 2–3 sets of each exercise. It doesn't have to be complicated and you can easily do it all at home. You can increase the load/weight/resistance over time as you get stronger. When you're exercising keep the movements slow and controlled and avoid rapid movements and any jerking.
- Avoid 'high impact' activities, such as jumping, running and hopping.
- Some activities that involve quick rotation or torsion – such as golf, or quick twists in yoga – may need to be modified or avoided, but this will depend on

the stage of your cancer, the location of the bone metastases, and whether or not you have pain or existing fractures. Speak to your doctor about this and make your own call depending on your individual circumstances.

- Avoid any activity which causes pain in the location of the bone metastases.

In summary, exercise (particularly resistance exercise) is extremely important for you if you have bone metastases or weak bones or are at risk of fracture. But unfortunately, most patients I come across have never been given this information. They are often given medication, but rarely advice on how to strengthen their bones. Seek advice from a specialist exercise cancer instructor or physiotherapist and try to keep as strong as you can.

I have a PICC line in my arm; can I exercise?

A PICC (peripherally inserted central catheter) line is a catheter in your arm which allows medication and fluid to be delivered into your body. It can stay in place for months and is convenient, preventing the need for frequent IV-line placement and cannulas. The line is usually stitched into place, so in most cases is secure and unlikely to come out. However, making sure the line doesn't become dislodged is a priority, along with taking care not to pull it out and being vigilant for infection. Keeping it clean and dry is important, and you should wear some sort of cover or sleeve over the top to protect it.

So, can you exercise with a PICC line in place?

This is an interesting question as there are no specific guidelines and each individual case is different, so you'll need to talk to your own doctor about your own personal situation. Most people seem to have no problem with most exercises – there are examples of patients who run, weight train, swim and continue as normal with a PICC line.

Walking, jogging or doing exercises involving the lower body, even weight training, squats, lunges and light weights using the upper body, all seem to be fine. Swimming may be possible if you can find a waterproof cover which makes your PICC watertight and prevents water or any sort of infection getting in.

It's generally thought that moderate exercise which doesn't involve too much repetitive upper body movement is perfectly safe for anyone with a PICC.

In fact, rather than being inactive, you do need to keep the arm moving as much as possible. Clotting can occur if your arm is immobilised or you're too sedentary.

Walking, jogging or cycling are all great exercise for general fitness. Safe exercises for the upper body could include using hand weights or a theraband – bicep curls, shoulder press and rowing-type exercises are all good. Light resistance and slow controlled repetitions of 8–12 reps each are fine. There are many people who exercise with a PICC without any restrictions, lifting heavy weights and doing upper body exercises with no problems at all.

Of course, if you see any sign of infection, swelling or pain at the PICC site, then see your doctor without delay.

I have a PORT; can I exercise?

A PORT differs from a PICC line in that the PORT is a central line inserted in the chest. It is used to deliver drugs, chemotherapy, fluids or nutrition directly into the body. The PORT reservoir is completely sealed under the skin and can stay in place for months and in some cases years. It doesn't need to be covered and people can go about their normal daily activities more easily. You can swim and there is no need to 'waterproof it' like you would do with a PICC.

In terms of exercise, once the incision has healed there shouldn't be any restrictions at all. Lifting weights, swimming, cycling and normal sporting activities such as golf are usually completely safe. If you're at risk of impact to the chest through boxing or contact sports, such as rugby or martial arts, or a fall from a horse, then please speak to your doctor or the person who placed the PORT to discuss any considerations.

I have peripheral neuropathy/poor balance; what should I do?

The most common neurological effect of cancer treatment is 'chemotherapy induced peripheral neuropathy' (CIPN). Although it's not fully understood, some chemotherapy drugs seem to cause damage to the nerves in the feet, toes, fingers and hands. It can result in numbness or reduced sensation, pain, burning or tingling. It can impair your balance or ability to grasp or hold items and increase the risk of falls if you have it in your feet. This is an area of growing research, and whilst currently there's no concrete evidence to suggest that exercise can improve or reduce the symptoms of CIPN specifically, it makes sense to keep moving to prevent general deconditioning, and some people do find their CIPN improves in time.

However, finding ways to be active is important for your overall health and cancer survival, as well as preventing muscle wastage and further balance/co-ordination problems.

Make sure you stay safe if you think you might fall or lose grip, so look at alternatives and structure any exercise programme to account for any loss of balance or grip issues. If walking is difficult, you may find using an exercise bike or swimming are better options. Specific seated exercises for lower and upper body strength can easily be done at home using hand weights or a theraband and are important to keep the muscles working.

If your feet are affected by CIPN, try simple exercises such as calf raises or sit-stand squats (holding on for support), and movements such as seated leg stretching, ankle rotations and mobility exercises to maintain movement in your feet and strength in your lower body.

I have a stoma; can I exercise?

Many people with bowel cancer will be given either a temporary or permanent stoma, so this is given a much more detailed overview in Chapter 4.

Key points

- There are surprisingly few absolute restrictions on physical activity when you have cancer. Everyone is different, will respond in different ways and will have different attitudes. There is no 'one size fits all' approach or set of rules.
- Remember that the benefits of being physically active generally outweigh any risks or potential harm.
- Whilst there are some guidelines for specific situations, these should be considered alongside your own personal situation and always get advice from your care team/doctor.
- Keep an eye on the bigger picture… especially your psychological wellbeing. Being active is incredibly important for our mental health and stress management. Weigh up your own reasons for being active against any possible risks.
- You might need to modify some activities, but generally you should be safe to do anything you want. You know your body best.
- Remember the subtle differences between 'exercise', 'physical activity' and

'movement' outlined in Chapter 1. There are very few situations where it's unsafe to 'move' and be 'physically active'. Walking, home-based mobility exercise etc, even at times when you might feel quite unwell, are safe and likely to help you feel better, not worse.

- Specific 'exercise' (going to the gym, running, playing sport), however, may require a different approach. You might need to modify more intense exercise routines or certain types of training during treatment or immediately post-op. Listen to your body and be flexible. Learn skills to modify, adapt and be creative.
- Try not to think about what you CAN'T do and think about what you CAN do instead. Find ways around challenges and barriers and find solutions/different ways of doing things.
- Try not to be fearful. What's the worst that could happen?
- And finally... remember that *something* is always possible. And *something* is always better than nothing.

Chapter 4

Living and exercising with a stoma

One of the most common questions from people who have had stoma surgery is 'Will I be able to exercise?' And the answer is 'Absolutely yes, you can!' and possibly more accurately 'Absolutely yes, you should!'

Other common questions include 'What exercise is safe?' and 'What abdominal exercises can I do?' and 'How can I avoid a hernia?'

These questions, and more, are the topic of this chapter and my area of special interest. I'm deeply passionate about helping people who have stomas become active and to overcome the many barriers and challenges.

What is a stoma?

The word 'stoma' means an artificial opening. A stoma is frequently required when you have colorectal surgery. It allows your bowel to heal after surgery, or is needed if your entire colon or rectum is removed. In this case, a stoma is formed by bringing a section of your bowel to the surface of your abdomen, through a hole in your abdominal wall. It is stitched into place and you wear a device known as a colostomy bag over the opening to collect the waste that comes out of your bowel.

Footnote: If you have a stoma, I recommend signing up for me+ - the patient support programme from ConvaTec. In particular, me+recovery is a specific stoma rehabilitation programme written and developed by me, available free of charge along with many other great resources from ConvaTec.co.uk.

The operations which create a stoma (sometimes just known as an 'ostomy') are of three types: a 'colostomy', an 'ileostomy' or a 'urostomy'. What's the difference between them?

- A **colostomy** is where the large intestine or colon is used to form the stoma. Colon = Colostomy. It is generally on the left-hand side of the abdomen (although not always). The waste that comes out of a colostomy is generally quite formed and resembles normal faeces. It's possible to irrigate the colostomy (flush out your bowel with water – this can be done at home) which provides much more freedom and means there's no need to wear a bag 24/7. Talk to your stoma nurse about whether this is possible for you. People who do this often say that it drastically improves their quality of life.
- An **ileostomy** on the other hand is a little different. It is formed from the terminal ileum at the end of the small intestine. Ileum = Ileostomy. An ileostomy is usually on the right-hand side of the abdomen. The waste that drains from an ileostomy can be very liquid and can resemble very loose stools or diarrhoea. This means your fluid losses are higher and you can be more at risk of dehydration, so people who have an ileostomy who are more active need to work harder at drinking fluids and electrolytic drinks. The bag itself will fill frequently and will need emptying numerous times per day.
- Occasionally people may need to have their bladder removed too, and this is where you have a bag to collect urine – known as a **urostomy**. This is more unusual in those with bowel cancer (although it does happen), so the focus of this chapter is on bowel stomas.

Some people will have a stoma for a short period of time while their bowel heals from surgery and it is then reversed. Once the bowel has healed (and typically when chemotherapy is over) they then go back to having their bowel re-connected.

Other people, particularly those who have a tumour in the lower part of the colon or the rectum, will have their stoma permanently. No-one knows the exact figure, but it's thought there are around 150,000 people in the UK with a stoma at any one time and it's becoming a more common procedure in people with bowel cancer.

If you're reading this awaiting surgery, you're probably feeling quite apprehensive. Your surgeon may be suggesting a temporary stoma, or you may already know that your stoma will be permanent. The most important thing I can tell you at this point, is that having a stoma is nowhere near as bad as it sounds. It truly isn't. I can tell you that, because I have one. I now run marathons and ultra-distance runs and live a perfectly normal life (see page 189 for 'My story').

Of course, it can take time to adjust, but once you do there are zero limitations to how you live your life. You can work, exercise, have sex, swim, travel, eat a normal diet and do any activities or job you wish without any limitations. There are many examples of athletes with stomas: mountaineers, world champion triathletes, cyclists, marathon runners and body builders who are thriving and living life to the full. There are also many people who have active jobs: tree surgeons, divers, police officers, fire fighters and doctors and nurses. There are also plenty of people who just enjoy normal activities such as dog walking, Pilates, jogging and dancing. They all find that having a stoma really isn't anywhere near as bad as they first thought.

It does not have to limit your life, and provided you have the right products and bag, there shouldn't be any problems or issues. No-one will know you have a stoma unless you tell them. The bags are incredibly discreet, and you can wear any clothes you like, including swimwear and sportswear.

What are the problems associated with having a stoma?

Unfortunately, we know from research that the vast majority of people who go through stoma surgery for colorectal cancer become *less* active than they were before their surgery. Ninety per cent of people with a stoma report not doing enough activity for good health (150 minutes per week of moderate intensity exercise). And many people never get back to being active. Their stoma and cancer treatment seem to become a permanent barrier (research awaiting publication).

This is a huge concern for many reasons. The negative effect on health in general and the risk of other chronic conditions (diabetes, heart disease etc.) by being physically inactive are significant. But on the flip side, people are missing out on so many benefits by *not* being active. As I have discussed in the past three chapters, exercise really is another form of treatment – it helps you feel better, recover faster, adapt to your stoma, improve your body image and boost your psychological wellbeing and quality of life. It's such an important tool.

Please don't let your stoma prevent you from being active. Living with a stoma is very much about adopting the right mindset. It might not always be easy, but maintaining perspective, finding solutions for problems and adopting a 'can do' attitude can be transformative in how you cope and adapt.

But there's so little information about exercise after stoma surgery that it's not surprising people are fearful and inactive. Surgeons, doctors and nurses often report that they don't know how to have an informed conversation about specific rehabilitation or exercise after stoma surgery. People are often left without information, guidance or support.

There are many issues often reported by people with stomas as 'barriers' to being active. Common ones are:

- other health conditions – arthritis, COPD etc
- lack of time
- family/work commitments
- pain
- lack of support and not knowing what to do
- not being given advice.

But these could apply to anyone regardless of whether they have a stoma or not. Specific 'stoma related' barriers appear to be:

- fear of parastomal hernia or symptoms from a diagnosed parastomal hernia
- dehydration – resulting in fatigue/weakness/lethargy
- leakage from the bag – or fear of leakage.

I'll now look at each of these in more detail.

What is a parastomal hernia?

A parastomal hernia is where additional loops of bowel push through the abdominal wall around the stoma and sit underneath the skin on the abdomen (see Figure 4.1). If you think about it, a stoma is itself a 'hernia' in the sense that a section of the bowel has been pulled through the abdominal wall. All we need to do as patients is minimise the risk of additional bowel coming through the opening, and try to reduce the risk of it getting bigger.

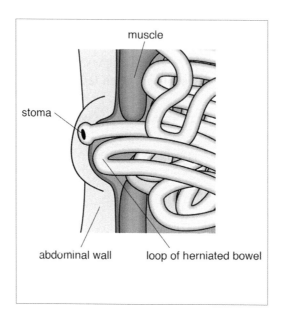

Figure 4.1 A parastomal hernia – a stoma with additional bowel protruding through the adjacent abdominal wall

Fear of getting a parastomal hernia is one of the most commonly cited concerns for people who have a stoma. And this is a real and genuine issue. No-one knows for sure, but it's estimated that anywhere between 50 and 70% of people with a stoma will go on to develop a hernia around it.[1]

The problem with a parastomal hernia is it can lead to problems with securing the bag and can increase the risk of leakage. It can cause more serious blockages and twisting of the bowel, as well as discomfort and body image concerns in those with larger, visible hernias.

However, it seems that this 'fear' of developing a hernia stops people from living life, from lifting things, from exercising and being active. In people who have already developed a hernia, the fear of it getting worse can be paralysing, leading to a very inactive and sedentary lifestyle. There is a tendency to catastrophise 'parastomal hernia', which leads to fear.

We know from research that the majority of people who do develop hernias actually report no problems, side-effects or issues at all. They say that whilst they know – or suspect – they have a hernia, it's not problematic.

So perhaps a hernia isn't always the big problem we are led to believe that it is. Of course, there are some hernias which are very limiting, uncomfortable and difficult to cope with, and these may well need surgical intervention, but for many people it may be better to put this worry to the back of their mind and continue life as normal.

Research into parastomal hernia prevention is ongoing, but at the moment no-one knows for sure how we can prevent them. There are lots of studies looking at the different variables and possible solutions – surgical techniques or non-surgical patient interventions. But the answer is probably that it needs to be a holistic patient-centred approach, combined with surgical techniques. As with everything there is no simple solution.

From an exercise perspective, however, we need to look at two things. One, what you can do as a patient to reduce your risk of developing a hernia, and two, what you can do if you already have one.

How to reduce the risk of parastomal hernias

According to the Association of Stoma Care Nurses (ASCN)[2] there are a number of risk factors which might increase your risk of developing a hernia. These include a wide range of surgical, medical and lifestyle risk factors.

There are things you can't do anything about such as:
- surgical techniques/number of surgeries/type of surgery
- medical conditions leading to your stoma
- other medications (steroids, for example) which may increase risk
- other medical conditions, such as diabetes, COPD and asthma
- having emergency surgery
- age – the older you are, the higher your risk.

And then there are lifestyle variables which increase your risk, and which you *can* do something about:
- being overweight or having a large abdominal girth (over 100 cm in particular)
- smoking – smokers are four times more likely to develop a hernia
- uncontrolled coughing due to COPD or asthma
- having weak abdominal muscles
- being generally deconditioned and unfit
- lifting heavy items with poor technique, which creates undue strain and force.

It's ironic that physical activity is often seen to cause damage and strain, increasing risk of hernia, when in fact the opposite is true. Staying as fit, strong and healthy as possible is more likely to reduce your risk of hernia.

To reduce your risk of hernia follow these basic guidelines:

- Keep your weight in check and stay as lean as possible.
- Keep your abdominal girth below 100 cm (39 inches).
- Avoid smoking, and if you do smoke, then make it a priority to give up.
- Ensure you treat a cough and keep asthma well controlled.
- Follow a 'core restoration' programme of exercises (see Chapter 7) after surgery, or pick it up any time in the future.
- Continue to strengthen all your core muscles, including pelvic floor, abdominal wall and back – and continue to do this for the rest of your life (Chapter 8).
- Learn how to lift correctly with good technique (Chapter 3), keeping items close to your body, and think about how you lift or move awkward items. Breathe out as you lift.
- Keep the muscles in your limbs strong so they can do the work when you lift and move.
- Practise specific breathing exercises (Chapter 7), and always breathe consciously during core and conditioning exercises – so your diaphragm works as part of your core.
- If you go to the gym or do other sporting activities, you will need to strengthen your core first with a gentle restoration programme to build foundations, then progress slowly back to your usual activities.

The importance of intra-abdominal pressure (IAP)

The concept of regulating 'intra-abdominal pressure' (IAP) is vital in reducing your risk of hernia. Learn how to move and lift things in a way which doesn't cause excessive IAP.

- Use your breathing – exhaling on exertion and not holding your breath are both useful things to remember.
- Avoid movements (lifestyle or sport-related) which involve bracing, static holds with heavy weights and pushing or pulling heavy or awkward items.

You'll know you've created excessive IAP if you feel your abdomen is 'doming' or you can feel (or see) a sense of pressure or increased bulging. If you get this sensation, then stop the exercise or activity you're doing and modify it, or adapt so you reduce the pressure. Your posture, breathing and the positioning of your body in relation to the item you're lifting all contribute and can influence IAP.

Do support garments help with hernias?

Some stoma nurses and surgeons recommend that people with a stoma wear a support garment, like a girdle, supportive pants/vest or a wide stoma belt, sometimes also called a 'hernia belt'.

These garments may help to support the abdominal muscles after surgery; however, the evidence on whether wearing one will reduce your risk of hernia isn't conclusive. At the moment we can't say that wearing a support garment will help prevent a hernia.

Wearing a garment for comfort, support for the bag and a smooth line under clothing can be helpful, however, and can improve quality of life and confidence. At the same time, support wear is not a substitute for strong and functional core muscles, and you can't rely on it to prevent hernia.

You need to strengthen your 'internal support garment' – i.e. the muscles of your core, including your pelvic floor – to improve function of the whole pelvic area and to get the muscles of your core working in synergy. Think about strengthening from within.

If you already have a hernia, then you may feel you need to wear some sort of garment, pants or a belt to provide some support and for comfort. Speak to your stoma nurse about what's right for you.

Can I exercise if I already have a hernia?

The answers to this question are the same: 'Yes, you can!' And 'Yes, you must!'. The hernia is only in one part of you; the rest of your body still needs to be exercised and kept mobile, fit and strong. It's very likely that keeping your weight down (or losing weight) and maintaining a functional core could prevent your hernia getting bigger or symptomatic.

However, we do know that people who already have a hernia feel apprehensive and nervous about being active in case they make their hernia worse. We know from research that people say having a hernia is hard to deal with; it lowers their quality of life. We also know that people become very inactive – scared to exercise and move.

Follow the same basic guidelines as for 'reducing the risk of hernia' (page 43) and pay particular attention to the concept of IAP – modifying movements and any exercises which might cause excessive abdominal pressure.

The core restoration exercises in Chapter 7 will be most appropriate; then progress to the exercises in Chapter 8, but please do speak to your surgeon (or a good physio) first if you have concerns.

However, if you've got an existing hernia it's wise to avoid exercises that involve lying face down/on your front (prone) – particularly 'bracing' movements, such as press-ups, planks, all fours and roll-outs, where the pressure will be forced downwards and into your hernia.

Instead, stick to exercises where you are lying on your back (supine positions) and watch out for that feeling of 'abdominal doming' or pressure around your stoma. If you get it, then stop the activity/movement/position and adapt and modify so you reduce pressure.

When it comes to lifestyle activities, be aware of how you pull, push and lift things in and around the home, especially if you have to 'brace' or twist whilst doing it – such as pushing/pulling a powerful or heavy vacuum cleaner or manoeuvring a lawnmower around a corner. Keep items close to your body, try not to extend heavy things away from your body, use your breath (breathe out as you lift), and use your arms and legs to do the work rather than placing force through your core.

Otherwise, try to have the confidence to exercise normally. Walking, jogging, cycling and swimming are all great ways to be active as is anything you enjoy – dancing, Tai Chi or whatever else.

Dehydration

A common barrier to being active is people finding they don't have enough energy and feel lethargic. If you're having cancer treatment it can be hard to untangle symptoms from side-effects, so speak to your care team or doctor to investigate and have tests done. However, it makes sense to eliminate as many potential reasons for fatigue as possible (such as anaemia) and work on the things that are within your control.

It's very common to become dehydrated if you have an ileostomy (less so with a colostomy). If it's also combined with chemotherapy, nausea, vomiting and low appetite/difficulty drinking, dehydration could easily become a big problem, and even land you back in hospital. Dehydration is covered in more detail in Chapter 9 (page 165), so please refer to that for specific information.

However, it's worth repeating a quick summary here too. The symptoms of mild but chronic dehydration include fatigue, lethargy and feeling 'groggy' – if you're feeling like this, don't just assume it's the norm or the fact you have a stoma.

You shouldn't have to accept feeling fatigued and lethargic. Good hydration is one of the 'quick fixes' that can instantly make a difference. See how you feel if you increase your fluid intake and drink more electrolyte drinks. Dehydration (and associated fatigue) shouldn't be a barrier to you being able to exercise.

One final important note worth repeating: if you have an ileostomy, don't just drink plain water. You need a mixed fluid intake (tea, coffee, juice, squash, milk and water) and it is especially important to include a daily electrolyte drink – which has the right balance of salts and glucose.

Drinking lots of plain water can flush the electrolytes out of your body and create a condition known as 'hyponatraemia', so keep your plain water intake to a minimum. Avoid sugary sports drinks (such as Lucozade) and instead have Dioralyte or SOS rehydrate, or make your own with a pinch of salt added to squash. Drink this daily to prevent dehydration occurring in the first place.

If fatigue continues or is particularly difficult, then speak to your care team.

Leakage/fear of leakage

And finally, I'll just touch on the third common barrier. Leakage from the stoma bag is a real concern for many people and the fear of having a leak can prevent them from going out, taking part in activities and enjoying life as they did before.

The topic of leakage is beyond the scope of this book, but all I'll say is that leaks are not inevitable or acceptable. There are literally hundreds of different types of bag, products and application methods and there will always be a solution. Do not suffer leaks or accept them as the norm. Speak to your stoma nurse for advice or call around the stoma bag manufacturers and ask for samples to try. We are so lucky that manufacturers are constantly developing and evolving new products, so keep trying until you find one that works for you.

Perhaps you're not suffering from regular leaks, but you worry that it might happen if you do exercise, sweat or go swimming? Then there are lots of tips and tricks to help you build your confidence. If you want to try going swimming but don't feel confident, test out the adhesion of the bag in a bath at home first. Check the bag in the water and see how secure it feels. Are your fears warranted? It's natural to worry, but stoma bags do create a waterproof seal and should be fine in water, even for many hours. The next step might be a short 10-minute swim at your local pool at a quiet time. It's all about building up confidence in your bag and system.

Sports and activities with a stoma

This section covers specific sports and activities in more detail and is aimed at people who are active or wanting to return to/take up a specific sport and who have a stoma. There are generally no limitations to what you can do when you have a stoma, but initially there may be a few considerations as you return to sports and activities. It's not quite as simple as just 'build up slowly' which is often the advice given.

You will need to go back to basics, imagine you're a beginner again and lower your expectations initially. A good rule of thumb for a starting point is to reduce your volume/intensity and duration by half (of what you were doing before), or by 75% if you've been very unwell for a long time. Watch out for movements or activities which create excessive intra-abdominal pressure, and listen to your body.

Colostomy UK also have a great leaflet covering all sorts of sports and activities with some top tips and advice.[3]

My guidelines for returning to exercise after stoma surgery are set out in Figure 4.2.

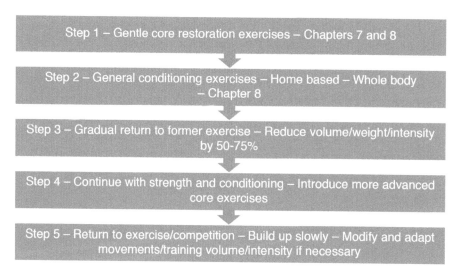

Figure 4.2 Five-step guide to returning to exercise after stoma surgery

You will also find some specific guidelines on modifying classic core exercises, such as the plank, crunches, leg lifts and bicycle, at the end of Chapter 8 (page 148).

Here are my top tips for some specific sports.

Running/jogging

- Running is a high impact sport, so pelvic floor and core exercises are super-important before you get started.
- After surgery, build up with a jog/walk plan even if you were a regular runner beforehand. If you're new to running, follow a beginner plan just like anyone else.
- Longer term work on the biomechanics of your core and whole body – stretching, foam rolling and strength work for your glutes (buttock muscles) and core.
- If you run longer distances, hydration will be an important consideration – take a bottle or backpack with you and use an electrolyte drink.

Cycling

- Initially start on a stationary bike or turbo trainer – build up confidence before you hit the trails/road.
- If you've had surgery to remove your rectum, saddle comfort may be a potential issue. Experiment with different types of saddle and use padded shorts. It may take a few months before you're ready to ride.
- If you need to lift your bike into the car or onto a rack, be careful with lifting overhead or awkward movements – take wheels off if you can, use a step to reach the roof of the car or a carrier on your tow bar which is lower.
- If you're a mountain biker, be conscious of how you lift and carry your bike on the trails – work harder on your core muscles before returning to trail riding.
- Have a good plan for hydration and nutrition on longer rides – use electrolyte drinks.

Swimming

- Get confident with the adhesion of your bag and choice of swimwear. There are lots of options so shop around. High street brands usually work just fine. A full body tri-suit works well for guys, or if you have your stoma above the waist.
- Work on your core exercises (Chapters 7 and 8) before you head to the pool

for the first time – swimming uses core muscles more than you think.

- Use a kickboard or pull buoy to begin with (kicking only or arms only – and alternate) and build up slowly with a modified/gentle stroke and only a few lengths at a time.
- Start with a few lengths – perhaps cut back by 50–70% for the first visit if you're a regular or competitive swimmer.
- Powerful strokes such as backstroke and front crawl have the potential to strain the abdomen the most and create high intra-abdominal pressure. Start with modified strokes/breaststroke and build up to front crawl gradually.

Tennis/badminton/squash

- Get fit with general conditioning, training off court first in the gym or at home.
- Practise at a tennis wall or squash court on your own in a controlled environment before you play a competitive match/knock up with a friend.
- All three sports involve impact, jumping and running, so work hard on your core/pelvic floor.
- Tennis has the potential to create the biggest strain and highest intra-abdominal pressure – so build up gradually to powerful serving.

Pilates/yoga

- Start with the 'core restoration' exercises in Chapters 7 and 8 before you start a Pilates class.
- Try a gentle post-natal-style Pilates or yoga class or online video as the postnatal-style approach is similar to rehab after surgery.
- Watch out for movements that increase intra-abdominal pressure, such as roll-downs, table top, straight leg raises (see page 146) – modify and adapt if you feel you're not strong enough or experience 'abdominal bulging'.
- Become expert at using your breathing – exhale on exertion and engage your core muscles.

Weight training/gym

- Strength training with weights/body weight is really important to combat age-related muscle loss and to maintain strength as you age. Don't be put off by worrying about lifting/hernia risk; the risk of complications from age-related muscle loss (known as sarcopenia) is probably far greater.

- Start with the 'core restoration' exercises in Chapters 7 and 8 to build your foundations first.
- Start with 'isolated' exercises for each muscle group (seated bicep curls, lateral raises etc.) initially and use lighter weights to start with. Seated exercises and machines might be a safer bet initially, rather than cables, free weights and big compound body weight exercises.
- In time you should be able to progress to most things in the gym, but always watch out for exercises or machines which create excessive intra-abdominal pressure – cables, pull-ups, planking etc.
- Ensure perfect lifting technique – use your breath. Breathe out on exertion/lift. Avoid breath holding. Get some coaching from a trainer to help.

Snow-sports/water-sports

- Start with the 'core restoration' exercises in Chapters 7 and 8 to build your foundations first.
- Then progress to more challenging core exercises. Snowboarding/ wakeboarding and skiing in particular need good core stability, so replicate the moves you'll do on the slopes in the gym or at home.
- Get fit away from the slopes/water with gym-based fitness training specific to skiing/snowboarding/water-skiing as you would if it was your first trip – include lots of core and leg strength work.
- Feeling confident with your bag and product choice is particularly important if you're out on the slopes or water and not close to a toilet. Make sure you have the product that works best for you and also find a waterproof dry bag to take your kit with you.

Golf

- Start with the 'core restoration' exercises in Chapters 7 and 8 to build your foundations first.
- Then progress to more challenging core exercises which involve rotation and replicate the 'golf swing' motion.

- Don't go back to a full round straight away. Try a few swings at the driving range first, then progress to nine holes.
- It can be helpful to use a buggy to begin with if it helps get you out, but don't rely on it in the long term. The walking is an important part of golf for your health!
- Take care with lifting and carrying the bag, particularly into the car or in and out of the buggy.
- Feeling confident with your stoma bag and product choice is particularly important if you're out on the course and not close to a toilet. Make sure you have the product that works best for you and keep trying samples until you find it.

Case study

Geoff had been told by his surgeon that he couldn't play golf again due to his stoma. For Geoff this was devastating, and he was really depressed. Not only was he a regular golfer, but Geoff was the Captain of the club and his house backed onto the course where he'd lived and played for over 20 years. He contacted me for an online consultation, wanting advice about whether this was correct and was there anything he could do so he could play again. Geoff's surgeon was being cautious and worried about potential twisting or rotation and the risk of hernia; however, for Geoff getting back to golf was a huge part of his recovery and the only thing that was important to him. It was clear that he would try anyway, so we needed to get him fit BEFORE he picked up a club! Initially I got Geoff working on core/abdominal exercises, which immediately gave him more confidence and feeling of core control. He worked on these exercises at home for around four weeks whilst also doing a 60-minute daily walk.

He then tentatively went along to the driving range where he gingerly took some gentle short swings. He only hit a few balls to begin with, but it was all fine and didn't cause him any problems. He continued doing his core exercises at home.

He then progressed to a full swing using his wood and practising three times per week, hitting more balls each time. Then after a few weeks he was able to get back on the course where he did nine holes. From there, he was able to get back to the club and do a full 18 holes around six weeks later. He made sure to use a buggy and avoided carrying his golf bag for long periods.

Geoff was delighted with this step-by-step approach which rebuilt his fitness and confidence gradually and allowed him to return to his beloved sport.

Contact sports/martial arts

- It's natural to worry about a blow to your stoma if you do contact sports or a martial art/boxing.
- There's no reason why you can't do any kind of contact sport or activity, and there are many examples of teams and individuals who play rugby or contact martial arts without any issues (see Colostomy UK for an example of their rugby team).
- Work on your core fitness and general conditioning for a few months before considering practice or playing a match. Then take a step-by-step approach and build up slowly, participating for only part of the match at first and gradually reintroducing yourself.
- You might want to consider a stoma protector (a bit like a plastic dome to cover the stoma) or some sort of padding in case you take a hit to the abdomen, but this is a personal choice and will depend on whether or not you feel it's a high risk. People generally start out with one for confidence but in time they realise they're not essential. Your stoma is actually very tough and resilient, capable of taking a knock or impact.

Finally, see References and resources (page 195) for details of my own stoma exercise rehabilitation programme me+recovery available from ConvaTec.

Key points

- There shouldn't be any limitations to what you can do with a stoma. You can swim, play rugby, do triathlons, marathons, hike up mountains and lift weights, or whatever you want. You may just want to make a few adaptations to help you overcome any barriers you face.
- Everyone who has had stoma surgery should do core restoration exercises (Chapter 7) after surgery, and progress to more advanced and whole-body conditioning exercises (Chapter 8) to restore core function after surgery.
- Those who were super-fit before surgery may try to dive straight back in to gym and fitness core exercises, but you must go through the core restoration programme first before hitting the gym. This encourages good core and pelvic function. Then progress to the harder stuff.
- Hydration is super-important for people with an ileostomy. Avoid plain water and instead have an electrolyte drink every day. Work hard on your hydration status to avoid fatigue and dehydration.
- Developing a parastomal hernia is a real risk for people with a stoma, but it's not a reason to be inactive and it's important not to catastrophise it. Watch out for excessive intra-abdominal pressure (IAP) and modify/adapt movements and activities if you feel pressure.
- Reducing the risk of parastomal hernia is multi-factorial and not just about doing core exercises or wearing a support belt. Work on all the factors within your control (smoking, coughing, weight control etc – see page 43) and do all you can to stack the odds in your favour.
- It takes time to adapt to life with a stoma, and some people find it very tough to come to terms with. But in time, you can and will lead a perfectly normal life. Use physical activity and exercise as a way to build your confidence and self-belief in what you can do, and don't allow your stoma to be a barrier to anything.

Chapter 5

Fatigue and self-care

Fatigue is the most commonly reported side-effect of cancer treatment, affecting around 70–100% of people with cancer.[1] It can be defined as a feeling of being completely worn out, weak, slow, without energy or having no 'get up and go'. Some people describe it as a deep exhaustion – just wanting to sleep and sleep and feeling unable to function. Cancer-related fatigue (CRF) is different from the fatigue people feel when they are otherwise well. 'Normal fatigue' in the 'non-cancer' population can usually be relieved by rest and sleep, after which you feel back to normal again.

Cancer-related fatigue is very different. People with cancer report that no amount of sleep or rest makes any difference and that it can last for months and even years. In some cases, it can affect their ability to take part in daily activities, relationships, socialising and day-to-day life. It can be really debilitating.

It's not a permanent state, however, and the severity of CRF seems to be dependent on where a person is with treatment, especially chemotherapy and radiotherapy.

There are some excellent online resources on cancer fatigue,[1,2,3] and I'd urge you to do some research and read up if you haven't already – see page 196 for full details.

What causes cancer-related fatigue?

There are many causes of CRF, and everyone is different. Not everyone experiences fatigue to the same degree and you can't predict how you might feel once you start treatment.

Try not to 'expect' to feel fatigued when you start treatment, and just wait to see how you respond instead. If you think you're going to experience fatigue, then you're more likely to. This is something called a 'nocebo effect'. In other words, if you're told you may have a negative side-effect, then you're more likely to look out for it, or attribute how you are feeling to the treatment or cancer.

But what exactly causes you to feel fatigued?

- Treatments such as chemotherapy, radiation, biological therapies and surgery can all cause fatigue in different ways. During treatment the body needs more energy to repair and heal tissue, and this appears to be one of the underlying reasons for fatigue. And there are many other cancer-related changes that can occur in the body, to your immune system and hormone levels, which can all contribute to fatigue.
- Anaemia – low levels of red blood cells in your body mean there is less oxygen – is a common cause of fatigue.
- Anxiety, stress and depression are common psychological causes of fatigue.
- Not sleeping well – because of pain, nausea, disturbed sleep, needing to use the toilet, anxiety, worry or insomnia – can all add to your fatigue.
- Other medicines can contribute to your fatigue.
- Other medical conditions, such as a heart condition, arthritis, diabetes or stroke, can cause fatigue on their own.
- Changes in your nutrition or hydration status – if you're finding it hard to eat and drink or are vomiting or aren't eating as much – can contribute to being fatigued.
- Being less active can actually make you feel more fatigued, although the reason why is not fully understood.
- The emotional strain of medical treatments, appointments and coping with your cancer diagnosis can be exhausting.

Some people report debilitating fatigue, while others have very little. Different treatments have different effects. Everyone responds in different ways and it can be really hard to unpick your symptoms and the reasons behind the fatigue.

Chemotherapy-related fatigue

People going through chemotherapy often feel the most fatigue in the days just after their treatment. The level of fatigue then tends to improve over the next couple of weeks, only to increase again with the next cycle of treatment. This gap can provide an opportunity to be more active and enjoy some normal quality of life before the next cycle begins. But try not to overdo it and end up on the 'boom and bust' cycle.

As the cycle goes on, fatigue can be accumulative, and many people say they feel most fatigued mid-way through their chemotherapy treatment. Some people also report that the feeling of fatigue continues when treatment is over and this can last for many years.

Radiotherapy-related fatigue

Fatigue due to radiotherapy is slightly different. As the treatment of radiotherapy doesn't generally involve a break, the fatigue tends to gradually build up so that by the end of treatment, people report being very tired. After treatment ends, fatigue generally stops, but it can take time to feel normal again. In some people, fatigue can last months or years.

Biological therapy/targeted therapy-related fatigue

Symptoms from biological therapies or targeted therapies vary depending on the type of therapy and how each person reacts to it. Some seem to cause some flu-like symptoms in some patients. People report feeling tired, having a fever, chills, muscle pains, headache and just feeling unwell. Others report very few side-effects at all.

Fatigue after surgery

It's normal to experience fatigue after major surgery anywhere on the body. Your body is healing, and it takes time to recover. Fatigue generally gets better over days and weeks as you recover from your surgery. But it can take many months, so give yourself time.

Other reasons for fatigue

There are lots of other reasons for fatigue and it can be hard to figure out what the causes are and what to do about it. If fatigue is a problem for you, then speak to your oncology team. They will assess your fatigue and may organise tests to identify any problems, and they can offer support and ideas on things you can do to help. They may suggest treatment for pain, or for anaemia such as a blood transfusion or nutritional supplement, or a change in medication, or counselling to help you manage depression or anxiety.

How can you treat fatigue?

Your oncology team will advise you how to treat your fatigue, so it's important to raise the issue as there are treatments to help if there is a clear reason for it.

Once you've ruled out or treated any physiological causes for your fatigue, or if it's become more chronic in nature, then it's time to put some strategies in place so you can help yourself. Think about this as 'self-care'. It applies to all of us, but when you're living with cancer or any other chronic condition, you need to pay much more attention to self-care strategies.

I work with many patients who have cancer, but also others who have chronic fatigue syndrome, over-training syndrome and heart conditions. Many of them suffer from fatigue and it can be debilitating and affect all areas of their lives. They regularly ride a red line between being able to live with a good quality of life, but then doing too much and falling into deep exhaustion. It can be very up-and-down and very frustrating. There's a very fine balance between getting enough rest but also getting moving and being energised.

Unfortunately there isn't a specific treatment for ongoing fatigue as such, and there isn't a simple solution. So, what does help?

You need to become an expert in YOUR own fatigue – What makes it better? What makes it worse? What can you do to help yourself? How can others help you? And then prioritise and work out strategies to help you manage it better.

Here are three key strategies to focus on.

1. Your energy bank – keeping it in balance. What drains you and what energises you?
2. Exercise – using exercise in a way to energise you rather than exhaust you.
3. Fatigue scale – keep notes, raise awareness and spot patterns.

It's a bit like piecing together a jigsaw puzzle. You need to work out the pieces you require and then start to put them in place. It might be challenging for you to do this, so ask for support from friends and family or your oncology nurse.

Your 'energy bank'

When you have cancer and are suffering from fatigue you need to prioritise the things that really matter to you. Your energy levels are limited and precious – like a rare commodity that you need to preserve. Just like a bank account for your money, imagine you have a bank account for your 'energy' and it's up to you to make sure it stays in the black. And just like when your money gets tight, you find smarter ways to spend and save, you need to do the same for your energy.

Grab some paper and a pen or make notes on your tablet, phone or computer. Whatever suits you best. Create two columns with the following headings:

Energy givers Things that give me energy	Energy drains Things that drain my energy

Think carefully about your current life and situation and about the 'drains' on your energy and the things that 'energise' you. These may not be immediately obvious, so give the problem some thought and come back to it in a day or so. Be thoughtful and reflective and really think about how you feel about each situation.

Here are some examples. Your table may be very different. Make your own list.

Energy givers Things that give me energy	Energy drains Things that drain my energy
Making sure I get to bed at 9pm every night	Shopping at the supermarket – really stressful!
Having dinner cooked for me by my partner	Getting up early to do the school run
Having a relaxing soak in the bath	Commuting to my workplace by train during rush hour
Going for a walk in the woods with my dog	Having a glass of wine at night – makes me feel terrible the next day

Spending time alone in peace and quiet	Having to attend coffee mornings and chat with people I don't really know
Pilates workout at home	Housework and preparing meals

Think about all the things you do in your life. Then assess if you feel they are an energy drain or an energy giver. Everyone will be different. Some things may be nothing to do with cancer. The difference is now you're depleted, your ability to tolerate the energy drains is much less.

Once you've identified some 'drains' and 'energisers', you can start to prioritise and work out strategies to make sure you have more of the left-hand column in your life and less of the right.

You may need to share this with your partner, family and friends and look at ways they can help you. If shopping at the supermarket is stressful and exhausting, can someone else do it for you? Or can you get an online delivery? Can someone help you with the school run in the morning? Instead of going to a coffee morning which you find stressful, just hook up with one friend for a calm chat at home. Can you ask your employer if you can work from home or work shorter hours?

This is not the time to soldier on. You need to put everything you can in place to help yourself. Where can you make life easier? Who can help you? Who's in your support team?

It's not always easy asking for help, especially if you're normally capable and on top of things. But try to think about it as keeping your bank balance in the black and freeing up your energy so you can focus on the things that really matter to you.

Exercise

To inspire you, Dr Mike Evans has a brilliant video online about cancer-related fatigue (CRF) and how exercise can help – highly recommended.[4]

Something that surprises most people is that rest and sleep do little to help cancer-related fatigue. It seems counterintuitive, but studies have shown that exercise (even tiny amounts) can actually help relieve fatigue rather than make it worse. The more you rest, ironically, the worse you will feel.

Exercise is one of the most beneficial ways to reduce cancer-related fatigue and should be seen as a method of treatment. Gentle aerobic exercise – walking, cycling, jogging etc – seems to have the biggest effect.

Being active, getting your blood and oxygen flowing around your body and working your muscles helps to give you more energy, not less. As you exercise, you also release 'feel good' hormones which make you feel better, boost your immune system and reduce feelings of fatigue.

And this is where my concept of 'intuitive movement' comes in (see Chapter 1). Find a way to move and be active that gives you energy rather than exhausts you. There's a very fine line between doing too much and doing just enough, and it can be hard to find out where that line is. Only you can do this, with trial and error and by what I call 'nibbling' away at exercise.

The 'nibble' approach

Try a small amount of activity – a 5-minute walk for example. See how you respond. If you feel okay and your fatigue isn't worse, next time take a slightly bigger nibble, try 6 or 7 minutes. Really small nibbles at a time!

If you were a regular exerciser before your cancer diagnosis, then you might want to have a rethink about your exercise levels and intensity. You may not be able to tolerate as much as you could before, and you'll require more recovery time after exercise. In time, however, you should be able to increase your exercise tolerance and return to your sport and activities.

Wherever you're at, the hardest part is getting started. Getting out of the door for a walk or making the conscious decision to go for a gentle run, swim or bike ride is often the most challenging barrier. But once you do, the chances are that you'll feel a million times better.

Fatigue scales

Try using a fatigue scale and diary to monitor your fatigue. Use a notebook or online journal – whichever you prefer – and each day I want you to score your fatigue level – morning, noon and evening at the same time each day. Also remember that during – and probably after – cancer treatment, there is no linear progression. Every day will be different. Some days you'll feel great, others you may not be able to get out of bed. So, you have to tune in to your body and listen to what it's telling you. Learn when to push yourself a bit, and equally when you really do need to take it easy.

You're looking for trends and patterns. Try to work out reasons why it may be better or worse than the previous day.

Use the following scale and, without thinking about it too much, just 'rate' your fatigue out of 10.

1	2	3	4	5	6	7	8	9	10
Extremely exhausted		Much fatigue		Moderate fatigue		Mild fatigue			Full of energy

Do the score 2–3 times per day and make a note in your diary or journal. How does it vary over the course of the day? Can you start to spot patterns in your fatigue from day to day? Or over the course of a week or a month? This may coincide with your chemotherapy treatment or days when you've been busy or not slept well. Make notes about your activities alongside so you can see how they are impacting your fatigue level.

If you're below 3 on the scale and feeling very fatigued, then it's probably best to rest completely. If you're moderately fatigued (4–5), then just try a 5–10-minute walk and see if you can boost your energy. Use your heartrate or a scale of 'exertion' to guide you (see Chapter 6). This will help you keep your intensity down and stop you pushing yourself too hard. Or see page 197 for details of a smartphone app for managing fatigue that you may like to try.

Now focus on the '3 Ps' to try and manage your fatigue better:

- planning
- pacing, and
- prioritising.

Planning

If you're on active treatment, it's critical that you plan fatigue management around your treatment. As chemotherapy and radiotherapy go on, your level of fatigue is likely to increase. You might need to plan for this and to expect it. After treatment has ended it may also take 2–3 months for your fatigue to reduce. In fact, it may continue to get worse. This surprises a lot of people who expect treatment to end and then to feel better.

So how can you plan? If you want to take a vacation – or have an important event to attend – can you plan it to coincide with a treatment cycle? How can you take advantage of the periods of feeling well between chemotherapy cycles? Can you use the opportunity to be a little more active or to enjoy a family dinner or trip?

Prioritising

This is the concept of the 'energy bank' and central to the self-care ethos. It's about being smarter with your time and energy and accepting where you're at right now.

When you have cancer, you will have less in the bank and lower reserves, so you have to prioritise activities, work and life events much more effectively. Think about the drains on your life and how can you manage them or reduce them. What is REALLY important in your life right now and how do you prioritise better? Don't be a superhero. Ask for help and if it's offered, grab it and take it!

Pacing

The concept of pacing really just combines everything we've already talked about. It's about knowing where your limits are and avoiding the 'boom and bust' cycle.

Booming and busting is exactly as it sounds. This is where you do too much when you're feeling good but end up utterly exhausted the next day. Your tolerance is likely to be much lower than it was before, so you walk a very tight line between doing 'just enough' and 'too much'. Only you can find out where that is. Which is why planning and prioritising are so important.

This is especially true of exercise. Your tolerance won't be as high as it was before. Much smaller amounts of activity may be exhausting, and you'll need much more recovery time. Think about pressing the 'reset' button and modifying your exercise. Remember the nibble approach and think about lowering your expectations. If you could do a 5-mile run before diagnosis, you might find that's too much at the moment. Or at least for a while. Remember though, this is a temporary state and your CRF won't last forever.

All you can do is experiment and find out where your tolerance level lies. Just take your level right back to zero and start by building up in tiny amounts like a complete beginner.

Pacing requires a balance of skills. You need to be flexible, accepting, adaptable and patient. Learn to say 'no' and ask for help. Practising self-care and compassion isn't always easy. But at times when you're struggling, you need to do it most. It's not selfish, it's about doing what you need to help you cope.

> ## Case study
>
> One of my clients, Rachel (30 years old), had recovered from colon cancer. I didn't know her when she was going through treatment, but I asked her if she had exercised at that time. She said yes, she had tried to, but it had been a disaster. I was surprised to hear this and she told me how one day during chemotherapy she had felt quite well and decided to go to her usual 'body pump' class at the gym. Because she was feeling good, she pushed it hard. Although she managed to 'get through it', she ended up in bed for a week totally exhausted. Sadly, she then wrote all exercise off as a bad idea and did nothing more until she had finished her treatment.
>
> What was her mistake? Rachel needed something different and gentler during treatment and to adapt her training regime. What she did here was 'boom and bust'. She would have been better doing a gentle Pilates class or going for a short jog or swim instead. But I get how hard it is. Rachel desperately wanted to be 'normal' and to be able to do her usual activities. But what she needed to do was to be more accepting of the fact she was mid-chemo and adjust her activities.

Growth mindset

The concept of 'growth mindset' was developed by Carol Dweck, a professor of psychology at Stanford University in the USA.[5] It's about adopting a mindset which allows you to grow, learn and develop, and to cope better with challenges and difficulties. It's used widely in sport and education, but it also has a place in dealing with illness.

People with a fixed mindset (the opposite of a growth mindset) don't feel able to control or change their circumstances. They don't learn from mistakes and don't display confidence in coping with challenges. They might say things like 'Oh why has this happened to me?' 'I can't do anything to change it' 'I can't exercise because I'm sick' or 'There's nothing I can do'. They have a belief that they can't change what has happened to them and have no control over their situation. They see problems and difficulties as barriers, preventing them from doing things.

People who adopt a growth mindset believe they have the power to change their circumstances, to find their way around challenges and difficulties, identifying solutions to problems and learning from mistakes. They might say things like 'What can I do to help myself?' 'How can I do it differently?' 'I might not be able to run at the moment, but can I walk or cycle instead?'

Growth mindset is much more than just being more positive or having a 'positive mental attitude' (PMA). A PMA isn't always helpful, especially when you're struggling. There's nothing worse than being told 'to be positive' when you feel low and depressed. It doesn't help. It's okay to feel down and miserable some days. Acknowledge it, accept and don't beat yourself up for not being 'positive'.

Growth mindset is different. It's about acknowledging the challenges and issues, but being creative, thinking of ways to overcome hurdles and ways of doing things differently. Knowing that you have the skills, knowledge and attitude to overcome them.

It might not come easily, but the good news is that just by knowing about the concept of growth mindset, you can start to change how you think and behave.

Think about the way you respond to difficulties and challenges and the inner voice in your head. What is it saying to you?

Dealing with cancer, treatments and the outcomes is incredibly challenging, but having a growth mindset just might help you cope better and find ways around the difficulties.

Here are some examples of growth mindset vs. fixed mindset:

Fixed mindset thinking *Instead of...*	Growth mindset thinking *Try thinking...*
I can't make this any better	It might be difficult, but what can I do to help myself?
I can't cope	Who can I ask for help?
I give up	I'll try a different way next time
It's too hard	It will take time but I'll keep trying
Other people cope better than me	How can I learn from them?
Why has this happened to me?	This is challenging but I can overcome it

Fixed mindset thinking *Instead of...*	Growth mindset thinking *Try thinking...*
There's nothing I can do	There's always something I can do. How can I make it better?
Why should I bother?	What more can I do?
It's all going wrong	I'll learn from this
Other people should help me	I can ask for advice and work out what I need to help myself
I can't do it	What can I do?

This is just a brief introduction to the concept and doesn't replace any support you might get from a counsellor or therapist, and it's really just a small taster of a huge subject. But it is amazing how shifting your mindset can have a dramatic effect on how you cope and overcome challenges. Cancer is often the single biggest challenge people face in life, and you need to dig deep to find skills, attitudes and strategies to help you get through it.

Find out more about growth mindset online or by reading *Mindset* by Carol Dweck.[5]

Self-care

The concept of self-care is becoming more popular, but it's still challenging for many people. It's common to feel guilty or selfish about caring for yourself. You might always put others first and before your own needs. But self-care isn't selfish or wrong. It's vitally important at all times of life, but even more so during cancer treatment and beyond. The phrase 'you can't pour from an empty cup' couldn't be more true at this point. Meaning that you can't give anything to others if you're depleted yourself.

A great analogy is when we travel by plane. If there is an emergency, the air cabin staff always tell you to put your oxygen mask on first, before helping others. You need to care for yourself and be in good health before you can help other people. The same goes in everyday life and especially if you're sick yourself.

When you're dealing with cancer, self-care needs to become top priority, especially if you have family and work to consider too.

There are lots of ways you can implement some self-care strategies. Here are just a few:
- make sleep a priority – get to bed early
- focus on nutrition and hydration – eat and drink the right things (more about this in Chapter 9)
- banish guilt about self-care
- say 'no' to things that aren't priority for you or things that 'drain' your energy
- try meditation and mindfulness
- make time for rest, relaxation and 'energy giving' activities
- make exercise a priority
- ask for help and accept offers of help
- delegate to others – don't try to do it all!

I'll focus on just a few of these below.

Sleep

Most of us are sleep deprived and we don't give it the priority it deserves. We don't get enough of the restorative, restful sleep that we need to function well in life. Some experts feel we are gripped by a chronic sleep crisis which is impacting our health in many ways, including being the root cause of obesity and ill health. Chronic lack of sleep can have an impact on your mental wellbeing, causing depression and anxiety, as well as increase your risk of diabetes, high blood pressure and heart disease.

Our sleep habits, behaviours during the day, medications and what we choose to eat and drink all have a huge impact on our sleep.

Unsurprisingly, sleep problems are even more common in people with cancer, creating a vicious circle of tiredness, insomnia and increasing fatigue. In fact, the National Cancer Institute estimates that over 50% of people with cancer have trouble sleeping.[6]

If you're having difficulty sleeping, falling or staying asleep, then there are lots of things you can do to improve the situation. Accepting 'poor sleep' as the norm isn't okay, and some small changes can make a big difference.

Talking about sleep and resting might feel at odds with being active and moving more. But it's not. It's actually the foundation. Sleeping well will help you cope, give you more energy and enable you to be more active and enjoy the benefits of exercise. And vice versa. Exercise can help you sleep better and improve the quality of your sleep – promoting deep REM (rapid eye movement) sleep.

Getting good sleep lowers your stress hormones, boosts immune function, reduces inflammation and promotes healing – everything you need when you're dealing with cancer.

There are two different aspects of sleep to focus on:

1. Getting enough sleep, in terms of hours – most people generally need around 7–8 hours of sleep per night.
2. Getting enough QUALITY sleep. This is slightly different. We need periods of deep sleep during the sleep cycle, so just being in bed for 8 hours isn't enough. We need both quality and quantity.

Sleep problems that can occur during cancer treatment (and beyond) include insomnia (due to worry and anxiety) and other symptoms such as night sweats, pain, nausea, side-effects of treatment and needing to use the toilet during the night.

Firstly, talk to you doctor or nurse about any medications that might be affecting your sleep and if there are any clinical investigations, pain management interventions or treatments you may need. However, alongside that, there is so much you can do to help yourself to boost your sleep.

Making it a priority is the first step. Accept that it's important and how much better you could feel if you felt more energised. Your body needs as much help as it can get right now… so try to create an environment for it to heal and repair, and sleep is a huge part of that.

The term 'sleep hygiene' refers to the behaviours/habits we have around bedtime, daytime activities, and our bedroom environment to enable us to get to sleep, stay asleep and get enough restorative sleep. Here are some 'sleep hygiene' tips that might help:

1. It sounds obvious, but have a regular bedtime. Make it a priority to be in bed at a set time each night. Work backwards from your bedtime to incorporate time for your evening meal, TV, reading, walking the dog and locking up the house etc. It's easy to get distracted. Set a time and stick to it.
2. Being more active during the day helps you sleep more deeply. Strength training exercises seem to be particularly effective, but make sure you don't exercise too close to bedtime as it can have the opposite effect. Try to exercise earlier on in the day instead if you can.
3. Make sure your bedroom temperature is right – not too hot or too cold. Open a window or have fewer covers. Choose natural fibres – cotton or bamboo

– for bedding and sleepwear which is more breathable. Try having a cool shower before bed which can lower your body temperature, especially if you get overheated in bed. Alternatively, a warm bath may be relaxing – see what works for you.

4. How noisy is your bedroom? Outside or in the room next door? Does your partner snore? Earplugs can make a huge difference if your sleep is disturbed by noise. There's a wide choice on the market – see page 197 for my recommendations.

5. Avoiding caffeine, sugar and alcohol before bed can make a real difference and it's worth keeping a diary of your food and drink intake so you can monitor symptoms and responses. Some people find they need to have decaffeinated tea and coffee. Alcohol seems to have a significant impact on quality of sleep, although you may not be aware of how it's affecting you. Alcohol can help you get off to sleep initially, but you're more likely to have disturbed restless sleep or wake up after only a few hours. When you need to get the best sleep you can, cutting out alcohol is probably one area where you can make an instant and positive impact.

6. It's well known that using a screen, mobile phone or tablet, or playing a video game, before bed can affect your sleep, but it's hard in our modern lives to avoid it. Watching a bright screen suppresses the release of melatonin – the hormone needed to help you get to sleep. If melatonin is suppressed, there is a disruption in the sleep cycle which not only affects your sleep on that particular night, but over time will affect your health. The best solution is to turn off your phone, tablet and screen at least two hours before bed. At the very least add a blue light filter to your screen or phone. Or just read a book instead.

If you're really struggling, talk to your GP about medication or counselling. A talking therapy known as CBT (cognitive behaviour therapy) has been shown to be especially useful in dealing with sleep problems, so it could be an avenue worth exploring or asking for a referral.

You could also consider trying wearable sleep trackers if you like gadgets and data – see page 197 for my recommendations.

Mindfulness and meditation

The concept of mindfulness and the practise of mindful meditation have been well studied in people with cancer.[7] There are enormous benefits and research has shown that people participating in mindfulness programmes have significantly less mood disturbance.

Mindfulness is a mind-body approach to life. It helps us relate differently to experiences and pay attention to thoughts and feelings. Regular mindfulness practice regulates the sympathetic nervous system and stimulates the relaxation response of the body, resulting in less chronic inflammation, less stress and fewer psychological symptoms.

Some of the most challenging aspects of cancer – fear, uncertainty, loss of routine and predictability – are well suited to mindfulness practice. Being in the moment can help us cope with our current situation better, focusing on what we can control in the present moment rather than worrying about the past or the future. It's thought to be a very compassionate, powerful and positive approach.

There are lots of ways to be mindful and there is a real cross-over with yoga and Pilates practice.

Repetitive activity such as swimming, running and walking – if done mindfully, without distraction – is just as good. Mindfulness can also be done more specifically as a meditation, which you can do with others by participating in a class or online group, or on your own using an app on your phone or downloading something to listen to (see page 197 for some suggestions). There are lots of resources for mindfulness practice if you look and you're sure to find something to suit you.

Mindfulness practice doesn't have to take much time at all. Start with 2–3 minutes at a time doing some simple breathing exercises.

Key points

- Fatigue is experienced by almost all cancer patients – some estimate as many as 70–80% of people who have chemotherapy or radiotherapy.[1]
- Although it may seem counter-intuitive, doing some physical activity or gentle exercise is the best antidote for cancer-related fatigue (CRF). Exercise is energising at the right volume and intensity (see pages 82-84). Get the balance right. Just enough to energise you, but not so much that you're tired out.
- However, try not to 'expect' to feel fatigued. This is known as the 'nocebo' effect. If you're told you'll experience a negative side-effect, then you're more likely to look for it or attribute it to your treatment or cancer. Instead,

keep an open mind and see how your body responds and tune into how you feel.

- Avoid 'booming and busting'. This is where you feel a bit better one day, then do too much, ending up exhausted and more tired than you were before. Instead, try to maintain consistency and regular activity. Little and often and small regular amounts is the goal. Hold yourself back on days when you feel great, and equally, give yourself a little push on days when you're struggling.
- Monitor your fatigue and energy levels using a numerical scale. This will help you spot patterns and trends and learn what to do about them. Having evidence that you feel more energised after doing some exercise is likely to help keep you motivated.
- Manage your 'energy bank' account by identifying drains on your resources. Work out what drains you and what energises you, then prioritise more of the 'energy givers' and find ways to avoid the drains. It might not be immediately obvious – sometimes activities we think should drain us are actually the things that energise us – so give it some careful thought.
- Make 'self-care' a priority. Don't over-commit to things. Only focus on the activities you really want to do. Delegate or put off tasks or activities that tire you or detract from your wellbeing.
- Quality sleep is essential. Make bedtime non-negotiable and practise good sleep hygiene. Sleep and exercise are interconnected. The more you sleep and feel more energised, the more likely you are to exercise, and vice versa. Exercise can improve your sleep quality, in particular deep REM sleep.
- Practise mindfulness – either specifically with a class or app, or indirectly through an activity which promotes mindful movement, such as walking, swimming, running or yoga.
- Develop a 'growth mindset'. This is much more than just 'being positive' and having a positive mental attitude. It is about focusing on what you CAN do rather than what you CAN'T. It's about finding solutions to problems and seeing ways to overcome hurdles, alternative ways to adapt and cope with situations. Having a growth mindset can be a powerful tool to help you as you navigate your cancer treatment.

PART III

THE EXERCISES

Chapter 6

Principles of exercise and monitoring

This chapter is about the basic principles of exercise and some of the science behind various methods of activity. If you can get to grips with the science behind exercise prescription and the 'why', you'll feel more empowered to plan and structure your own activity.

Each of you reading this book will have different disease prognoses, treatments, outcomes, symptoms, exercise preferences, other medical conditions and relationships with exercise. And because of that, there is no one-size-fits-all approach. It's literally impossible to have a specific plan or programme that's right for everyone.

What I think is a better approach is for you to understand the basic principles of exercise; then you can structure, monitor and progress your own activity and response much more effectively.

So, let's look at four areas in more detail:

1. the current guidelines for physical activity when you have (or are recovering from) cancer (page 76)
2. the six components of fitness – muscle strength and endurance; body composition; balance; agility and co-ordination; flexibility; and cardiovascular fitness (page 77)
3. the FITT principles of exercise (frequency, intensity, type and time) (page 82)
4. heartrate monitoring (resting, training and recovery) and RPE (rating of perceived exertion) (page 84).

Guidelines for physical activity when you have (or are recovering from) cancer

There are two sets of guidelines that you need to be aware of. First, the World Health Organization (WHO) guidelines for the general population[1] apply to you if you are recovering from cancer and have completed your treatment. These guidelines state that all adults should aim for the following each week: (1) 150 minutes of moderate physical activity (ideally spread out throughout the week in blocks of 10 minutes or more); (2) also two sessions of muscle-strength promoting exercise (this can be specific resistance exercises with bands, weights or body weight or less formal lifestyle activity such as DIY, gardening or housework).

Second, the American College of Sports Medicine (ACSM) published guidelines in 2019[2] for people currently undergoing treatment for cancer or those with symptoms. These guidelines recommend a little less each week – aiming for around 30 minutes of physical activity three times per week. This may feel a little more doable and realistic.

What does that mean for you?

Moderate physical activity is where you get a bit out of breath and your heartrate increases. This is vital for cardiovascular (heart and lung) fitness and to get the benefits of exercise for heart health. But it doesn't mean you have to be gasping for breath, red in the face and working at your maximum. Brisk walking will do the trick, but you do need to do it at a pace that gets you slightly out of breath. Around 3 mph is considered a reasonable pace.

See page 197 for details of an NHS app for your smartphone to help you achieve this.

The target of 150 minutes spread over the week can be broken up into 20 minutes x 7 days of the week or 30 minutes x 5 days of the week. Ideally, not all 150 minutes in one go. Little and often is the best approach and you can also break it up further into 10-minute blocks. A 10-minute block is thought to be the minimum requirement for health benefits.

There is also a dose response. This basically means that the more you do the greater the benefits. The 150 minutes is really a minimum target.

For people with cancer, even those on active treatment, the recommendations are exactly the same. Aim for 150 minutes of moderate activity per week and two strength sessions. This surprises a lot of people – especially some doctors and nurses who are unaware of the guidelines, and also patients who think that they should rest.

The second part of the recommendation is less well known, but I actually think it is equally, if not more, important. Muscle-strength-promoting exercise or strength training should be done at least twice per week. We know that very few people manage to achieve this. Yet it doesn't have to be as difficult as you think. Again, the little and often approach is the best way to tackle it.

Maintaining our muscle mass – especially when we get older/during illness/after surgery – should be an absolute priority. Muscle-strength-promoting exercise involves working against some sort of resistance to build muscle strength, or in many cases just to prevent muscle loss.

This doesn't have to be weight-lifting in the gym – although that's great if you can do it – anything where you use your muscles against resistance is good. Using exercise bands or small hand weights at home, or doing things like squats or push-ups using your own body weight, are great. But equally, lifestyle activities such as DIY, gardening and housework, especially if you're lifting, carrying, pushing and pulling, will all help keep your muscles strong. Government recommendations[1] suggest we do at least two sessions per week of exercise which strengthens muscles to prevent age-related muscle loss.

There are a whole host of complex social, physical, economic and psychological reasons why people don't achieve these targets and I know just how hard it is.

So, if you're struggling to get anywhere near these guidelines, then don't be discouraged. Anything is better than nothing. Getting motivated to just get moving a bit more, do something and get started is great. Be proud of your achievements and learn to be 'okay' with where you are at right now.

Six components of fitness

What does 'fitness' mean to you? The chances are it means different things to each of you reading this book. Being 'fit' really means being 'fit for purpose'. That 'purpose' will be different for everyone. It might be running a marathon, competing in ballroom dancing or simply being able to go back to work, or to walk to the shops for your paper.

There are essentially six key components to physical fitness – see Figure 6.1.

These six components are all interconnected and important for basic daily functions, such as getting in and out of a chair or bed, walking, sitting upright, climbing stairs, lifting and carrying things, doing shopping, driving and so on. This is known as 'functional fitness', and for many people during cancer treatment and afterwards that's the first goal.

And then as we become fitter, these components interconnect to help us be more

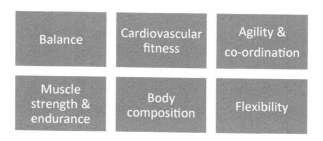

Figure 6.1 Components of fitness for health

active, to participate in sport/exercise or vigorous lifestyle activities and to reduce our risk of injury. We need balance and flexibility when walking or running, to have the arm power to swim or dig the garden, to have leg strength to cycle or squat. To be flexible enough to lunge for a ball and to have agility to move around the court to play badminton or tennis or play with children.

Each component is important, but, depending on what we are doing, some more than others. If we look at athletes, different sports will need different priorities. Balance and agility are a focus for a ballet dancer or a gymnast, whereas cardiovascular fitness is more of a priority for a marathon runner or a rower.

For basic daily functioning (to enable daily living, dressing/washing, shopping, work, housework and avoiding falls etc), we need all six components of fitness. Some of the first signs of muscle loss are when you find it hard to push yourself up out of the bath (muscle weakness in the upper body) or when you find that you 'plop' yourself down on a chair heavily. This means your leg muscles aren't strong enough to control the lowering of your body weight.

An indication of lost flexibility (in your shoulders) is when you can't fasten your bra or do up a zip at the back of a dress or top. And loss of balance might mean you trip easily, feel unsteady on your feet or find you're not able to stand on one leg to tie your shoe laces. Watch out for any of these signs and then do something about it before it's too late.

When we are ill, spend time in bed and/or hospital or have surgery or cancer treatment, all of these components will be affected. It's that feeling of being weak, out of condition, struggling with everyday activities and just feeling vulnerable and mistrusting your body.

I'll now focus on the components in Figure 6.1 in more detail. 'Cardiovascular fitness' refers to how well your heart and lungs are functioning. Exercising at 'moderate intensity' will have health benefits for your heart and lungs – more on this on pages 82-90.

Muscle strength and endurance

The old saying 'if you don't use it, you lose it' applies to muscle tissue probably more than any other part of you. Being inactive for long periods of time can cause extensive muscle loss. If you've ever broken an arm or leg and been in a plaster cast, you'll know exactly what I mean. The limb that has been immobilised rapidly becomes thinner and smaller after only a few weeks in the cast. The muscle basically wastes away when it's not used. In a nutshell, this is muscle loss, something we call 'atrophy'.

Our bodies are made up of various components, including muscle, fat, bones and organs. Muscle makes up around 30–40% of our body. Muscles attach to bones to keep us upright, help with balance, help us move, lift, carry things, get in and out of chairs and bed, climb stairs and keep us strong and mobile.

Strong muscles impact balance and joints and prevent us from falling and developing arthritis. Maintaining muscle mass as we age should be top of our priority list. One important aspect of muscle which isn't as well known, however, is its role in controlling blood glucose levels in the body. The more muscle we have, the better our bodies are at regulating blood glucose. This means that strength exercises have important implications in the prevention and management of diabetes. Simply put, we all need strong muscles for our health, no matter our age or lifestyle.

Age-related muscle loss

As we age, we lose muscle at approximately 1% per year, which doesn't sound too bad, until you add it up over a couple of decades.

This 'age-related' muscle loss is known as sarcopenia and, contrary to popular belief, it's not inevitable. Any kind of 'strength-promoting exercise' is vital as we get older to prevent this muscle loss and why the government guidelines suggest two sessions per week of 'strength exercises' in addition to the 150 minutes of cardiovascular exercise.

The older you are, the faster you lose muscle when you're in hospital. It's well known that 10 days in a hospital bed can cause up to 10% muscle loss in people over the age of 80. Frighteningly, this is equivalent to ageing by 10 years – effectively, turning an 80-year-old into a 90-year-old after only 10 days in hospital. This muscle loss can be devastating, causing patients to become immobile, frail and dependent in a very short time.

Illness-related muscle loss

Illness-related muscles loss is known as 'cachexia'. This is where there is some sort of metabolic disease or illness also present which causes the body to lose muscle even more rapidly. Your body is basically trying to fight the illness and needs to use every stored resource it has available.

Cachexia is very common in people with cancer, especially if you're undergoing chemotherapy. This is why we recommend you try to remain active during treatment and also to eat a diet high in protein foods which help to repair and rebuild muscles, or at the very least to prevent too much muscle loss.

It's possible to reduce some of the rapid muscle loss and decline, simply by doing some resistance moves. You can do this by doing the exercises in Chapter 7 to keep your legs and arms strong and just by trying to avoid inactivity as much as possible.

As well as walking, using stairs and just moving around more in daily life, there are specific exercises you can do at home using bands, weights or your body weight. For example, chair squats and calf raises for your legs and hand weights or resistance bands for your upper body. Weave exercises into your day – squats when waiting for the kettle to boil or calf raises when on the phone or watching TV. See Chapter 7 for more ideas.

For those who were already active before treatment, working out with heavier weights in a gym or at home is also a great idea – during treatment try 2–3 shorter sessions per week of 10–15 minutes. Little and often is probably best but be guided by how you feel. During treatment you might need to reduce the volume and weight from pre-cancer training (possibly by 50-75%) – although there are no real guidelines. You may also experience more muscle soreness, so factor in more recovery time and wait a day or so to see how you respond before doing more.

Get advice from a trainer or exercise specialist trained in cancer rehabilitation. You'll have slightly different goals depending on your treatment situation:

– **During treatment:** do what you can to minimise muscle loss. Don't expect to have muscle gains during treatment. Try higher reps of body weight or light weight training and just see what you can tolerate.

– **After treatment:** you can start to progress and see an increase in muscle development again, but be aware your tolerance of volume and weight may have changed, and you'll need more recovery. Nutrition and protein intake will be a super-important focus to aid muscle development. Be aware of your 'intra-abdominal pressure' (IAP) if you've had abdominal surgery and be cautious with very heavy lifting and certain core exercises. See Chapter 7 for core rehab exercises and Chapter 4 for more information on exercise with a stoma if that applies to you.

Body composition

The 'body composition' component overlaps with 'muscle strength'. Body weight taken in isolation (or BMI – body mass index) is not a true indicator of health status. In general, it's better for health to have more muscle and be stronger, which may mean being heavier. Being 'thin' or 'light' is not always a good thing if you're not active.

During cancer treatment it's common to experience body composition changes. You may lose muscle and become weaker, and your body composition may become altered in a negative way. However, some people find that they gain weight during cancer treatment, due to steroids, inactivity or changes in appetite and eating habits. This is often body fat rather than muscle.

So, whilst our body weight is important to a certain degree, our *body composition* is a far more useful way to measure how healthy we are. Ideally, we want to have more muscle and less body fat. Cancer treatments, surgery and chemotherapy can all make it hard to maintain healthy body composition. Which is where exercise comes in.

Your diet plays a big role in your body composition and how much muscle you have, and even more so during and after cancer treatment. Alongside being active, eating foods rich in protein, such as meat, fish, eggs, nuts, beans and dairy, is vital to help repair and regain muscle tissue. There's more on this in Chapter 9 Healthy nutrition and hydration.

Balance, co-ordination and agility

These three components are interconnected and similar but with distinct differences. All three components can be affected during cancer treatment, leaving you feeling unbalanced, at risk of falls and vulnerable.

When balance, co-ordination and agility are affected, it can make doing simple things, like walking over uneven ground or climbing stairs, more difficult. Daily living activities, such as getting dressed, putting on socks or shoes or getting in and out of the shower or bath, can become more challenging.

- **Balance** is defined as the ability to maintain a static position without falling or to move steadily over an uneven surface (dynamic balance).
- **Co-ordination** is the ability to use different parts of the body together, such as using your arms and legs together to walk briskly.

- **Agility** is defined as the ability to change direction quickly with control and is closely related to dynamic balance. An example of this would be being able to step out of the way of a car when crossing the road.

However, it's important to remember that all these components can be improved with the right exercises.

Feeling unsteady on your feet, weak or not able to do the things you could do before is not a good feeling. You're more likely to fall or to need walking aids. So please try to work hard to stay balanced, mobile and strong. It's surprising how little you have to do to make a difference. Try doing 5 chair squats and 10 calf raises 3 times each day and you'll soon see a huge change (see Chapter 7). Or simply stand on one leg withoug holding on, and see how long you can manage.

With time, persistence and practice, you can improve all of these components, but it doesn't happen without some work on your part. Don't give in to the feeling of 'vulnerability'... you CAN do something about it, and you will get stronger again.

Flexibility

Flexibility is defined as the ability to bend and stretch without injury or discomfort. Cancer treatments can all affect flexibility and generally make our muscles and joints feel stiff and tight. Being able to reach up to a high shelf or bend down and tie your shoelaces are good examples of needing flexibility in everyday life.

Generalised lack of flexibility is common after long periods of bed rest or inactivity. Muscle loss is linked with lack of flexibility, injury or pain. And this becomes a vicious circle. The more stiff and inflexible you feel, the more likely you are to injure a muscle or develop a joint problem.

So, to wrap up, ALL six components of fitness are important and interconnected. The exercises in Chapter 7 will help you work on all of them in different ways, helping you get stronger and more confident.

FITT principles of exercise

The FITT principles of exercise are a simple way to help guide and structure any exercise plan and during cancer treatment I think they are even more important.

- Frequency – how **often** you exercise or do an activity.

- Intensity – how **hard** you work – measured by heartrate or the weight you lift.
- Type – the **type** of activity or exercise (cycling, running, walking, Pilates etc).
- Time – how **long** you do it for.

Keeping it really simple, when you're thinking about being active or start to do more exercise, you only focus on ONE of the principles at any one time. If you try to increase all four at the same time, you'll end up injured, ill and exhausted.

The FITT principles guide us and ensure we build up exercise in a safe way. This is particularly important for anyone with cancer. You need to dial back your expectations and give your body much more time to recover and adapt.

So, when we are increasing the amount of activity we do, we need to take it step by step and work on the four FITT principles in a specific order. This approach applies whether you're already fit or a new exerciser.

1. **Frequency**: Little and often is the best approach to exercise and building up a regular habit is priority. Initially all you need to focus on is increasing how often you do something. If you walk twice per week at the moment, work on frequency first before changing anything else. Simply add another short walk per week, and then another, so eventually you're walking 4–5 times per week. The same goes if you run, go to the gym or swim. Regular, consistent exercise is the key as well as a gradual increase in frequency. Forget about how hard or how long you do it for initially, just think about bite-size snacks of movement throughout the day and the week. It's better to do 5 x 10 minutes of exercise per week than 1 x 50 minutes.

2. **Type**: As much variety as possible is the best approach. Think about the six components of fitness and try to find ways to cover them all. Mix things up with Pilates, walking, swimming, active housework, cycling and weights. If you're just getting started or currently on active treatment, a mix of movements from Chapters 7 and 8 of this book and some walking would be great.

3. **Time**: How long you do something for comes after you've built up a regular habit of bite-size chunks. Your exercise duration tolerance will be affected by your cancer treatment and you are likely to find that even short periods of exercise can be tiring. You may find you need to cut your duration of exercise down by 50–75% of previous levels. If you could run for 45 minutes before your diagnosis, you might only be able to manage 15 minutes now without being really fatigued. But that's okay! It's where you are right now that matters, and something is always better than nothing. Don't expect too much of yourself especially if you're still on active treatment or just had surgery. Use the 'nibble approach' to

build up exercise duration – add on 1–2 minutes each time to a walk, run or swim or session. Lower your expectations and see how your body responds before you add on any more time. Duration is the one component which can wear you down more than any other, so proceed gently. You may find that 10 minutes is enough, especially on days after chemotherapy or during radiotherapy.

4. **Intensity** comes last. This hooks into the 'intuitive' approach to exercise and is where many people go wrong – pushing themselves too hard to begin with or when feeling unwell. How 'hard' you exercise comes into focus only when everything else is in place. When you're able to exercise regularly, tolerate more duration and recover well, then you can start to think about increasing pace, speed or weights. How hard it FEELS to you is the only thing that matters. I advise people to keep the intensity of anything they do to a gentle level (feels like 5 on a scale of 1–10). You can get health benefits from moderate exercise, by just getting a little out of breath, but without pushing it too hard and exhausting yourself. Exercising too hard can put you off, and your brain will eventually find a way to stop you. Be kind to yourself and don't push it too hard too soon.

Heartrate monitoring

Monitoring your heartrate is a really clever way to exercise and get to know your body. I think it's one of the most simple but underrated ways to help you structure exercise, and get the best from your activities.

Knowing your heartrate at rest, during exercise and when recovering is really insightful and gives you great feedback. It doesn't have to be complicated at all, so don't be put off. It can help you monitor your progress and recovery and can provide a guide to when to exercise and when to rest.

In very basic terms, your heart is a muscle like any other in your body. Each beat pushes blood and oxygen around your body. And like any other muscle in your body, the goal with any cardiovascular exercise is to strengthen the heart muscle so it's more efficient. A bigger, stronger heart will pump more blood with each single beat. A small, weak heart will need to beat many more times to push the equivalent amount of blood around.

Resting heartrate (RHR)

Knowing your heartrate *at rest* (RHR) is important. The lower the number the more efficient your heart is, and the fitter you are. Monitoring your RHR over time gives you important information about your fitness – as you get fitter the number will come down. But also, if there are changes in your RHR it may mean you're unwell, not recovering or struggling with treatment – and therefore you can adjust your exercise (or rest) in response.

How to measure your RHR

Find your pulse either at your neck or wrist and count the number of beats for one minute. Time it accurately. Do this first thing in the morning, before you have coffee or tea or get up out of bed.

Record the measurement in beats per minute (bpm). It will be somewhere around 50–80 bpm.

Record it at the same time for three days, and then take the average.

You could also measure your RHR using an app on your phone or with a fitness tracker watch (see page 198 for details).

Things that can increase RHR include:

- caffeine
- dehydration
- alcohol
- fatigue
- stress/anxiety
- illness/infection
- certain medications
- losing fitness.

Things that can decrease RHR include:

- medication for heart conditions and blood pressure (beta blockers)
- getting fitter.

Monitor your RHR from time to time and keep an eye on the number over a period of weeks and months. Is it going up or down? If the number goes down, it's a sign of increasing efficiency and fitness.

If you measure your RHR and notice it's higher than usual, it can be a sign of fatigue or illness. If you notice an RHR which is 5–10 beats higher than your average, then it's an indication that your body is under stress for some reason. This is an indication NOT to exercise that day or to do a session which is very gentle – perhaps just some stretching or a walk.

Remember the 5–10 beat rule – if your resting pulse is 5–10 beats higher than normal you should take a day off, lower your training intensity or rest.

If it's much higher or lower than normal (below 40 or higher than 100), then check in with your GP, oncologist or nurse.

Exercise heartrate (EHR)

To measure your EHR you'll need to purchase a heartrate monitor with a chest strap or wrist sensor (see page 198 for recommended brands). This gives you realtime feedback about what your heartrate is doing and the intensity of your exercise. This is relevant whether you're just out walking or doing something more strenuous, such as hiking, cycling, swimming, jogging or doing an exercise class. And it's a really helpful tool as you're starting to 'reset' your exercise boundaries during and after cancer treatment.

Think back to the FITT principles and the importance of 'intensity' (page 83-4). Aiming for a 'moderate intensity' of exercise during or after cancer treatment is considered to be safe and appropriate. But how do you know what 'moderate intensity' is and how does it feel?

Measuring your heartrate as you exercise gives you a way to monitor exercise intensity and keep it at a 'moderate level'. It helps you to get the most from your exercise session but also ensures you don't overdo it – which is vital, especially during treatment or if you're really fatigued. It also helps to give you some structure to your exercise and to build your confidence as you can see what your heartrate does in response to picking up the pace or slowing down. Using heartrate means that your body is guiding the intensity, which is super-important when you're having treatment or you're on the road to recovery. You're learning to tune into your body and let it guide you.

For most people 'moderate intensity' will correspond to an EHR of around 70-75% of their maximum heartrate; that's around 115-145 bpm depending on their age (lower as one gets older). The idea is that you do your exercise at this figure – monitoring it on your watch or phone - keeping an eye on it and making sure it doesn't go too high. This will mean you're getting the benefits of activity but not overdoing it. However, the problem is that it's unlikely you'll know what your maximum heartrate is.

If you have a high-tech watch, it's possible that it will calculate an 'Exercise Heartrate Zone' for you based on the information you input when you set it up (usually using your age or date of birth). If so, you want to look at the zone which is 70-75% of your maximum. This will give you the right intensity to exercise at.

If you don't have a high tech watch, then all you need to do is work out your own EHR target using a simple formula. Luckily there is a simple way to do this – the Maffetone Method – which gives you a reasonable guide to stick too. We don't need to be too specific here – it corresponds well to exercising at a moderate intensity or at around 70-75% of your maximum. Use the following formula:

180 minus your age = target exercise heartrate (EHR)

So, for someone aged 50 years:

180 - 50 = 130 bpm.

So when exercising, aim for a heartrate of around 130 bpm (a zone of around 125-135 bpm would be fine). This gives you the all-important 'moderate intensity'. Not too low and not too high. The goal is to have this number (or a relatively tight zone) as a ceiling for the majority of any exercise you do. This means you're exercising at an aerobic level, enjoying the benefits of being more active, but not pushing yourself too hard.

Your EHR is never static, though; it fluctuates throughout a session. Walking up a hill will push it higher, for example. It is reasonable to aim for a range around your EHR target. In this example, 125–135 bpm would be a great goal, keeping 135 bpm as the absolute maximum. If it starts to go higher, drop the pace, slow down and allow it to come down.

This is not just for people with cancer; I use this formula with a lot of my clients. It helps them build good aerobic fitness without becoming too fatigued. And I think, for people with cancer, that has to be the priority and is possibly even more important. Don't be too specific though, and don't worry too much. You're just trying to find a zone to aim for to guide you to the right intensity. Work out your own numbers and start to monitor and see how you feel.

That said, I do know people with cancer who exercise much harder than this, and that's fine too if you feel well enough, have no symptoms which might indicate a cardiac issue and are at low risk of a cardiac complication.

Earlier guidelines for cancer patients used to suggest a low intensity of exercise (70% of maximum heartrate or less), but a more recent study[3] suggests that for people without cardiac complications or for those having chemotherapies not linked to cardiotoxicity, it may be safe to exercise at a higher intensity, if you feel up to it. And it's possible that there could be benefits for colorectal cancer patients, including reduced onset of fatigue and potential ability to tolerate treatment better. This is, however, a newer area of research and there is currently very little guidance about exercise intensity in people during or after treatment. So, if in doubt, maintain a lower heartrate and keep your exercise intensity gentle and below 70% of your max HR.

It's important to speak to your own oncologist about the type of treatment you've had, your risk of cardiac complications and exercise intensity, and to take their advice.

Be guided by your body and find the level of intensity that's right for you. Being able to exercise again the following day and maintain consistency is the goal – not being flat out in bed because you've overdone it. It's all about finding the right balance.

RPE – rating of perceived exertion

If you don't like the idea of a heartrate monitor or don't wish to purchase one, then using RPE is also a super-simple way to monitor exercise intensity. RPE stands for 'rating of perceived exertion' and is a reliable – yet simple – way to monitor how hard exercise feels to YOU at that moment – see Figure 6.2.

1	**Very light activity** (anything other than complete rest)
2-3	**Light activity** (feels like you can maintain for hours, easy to breathe and continue conversation)
4-5	**Moderate activity** (feels like you can exercise for reasonable periods of time, still able to talk short sentences but starting to feel out of breath and heartrate is increasing)
6-7	**Vigorous activity** (on the verge of becoming uncomfortable, feel short of breath but only just able to speak a sentence)
8-9	**Very hard activity** (difficult to maintain intensity, hard to speak more than a few words, feel out of breath)
10	**Maximum effort** (feels very hard, considerably out of breath, unable to talk, unable to continue)

Figure 6.2 RPE scale (rating of perceived exertion)

Aiming for 4–5 on the RPE scale for the majority of your exercise will give you the most benefits but isn't too hard. So, if you go for a walk – you need to be walking briskly enough to feel a little out of breath. At this level you should be able to chat, possibly even sing, without feeling too out of breath.

If you're feeling unwell, currently on treatment or very fatigued, remember that something is better than nothing. Even if you just get to 2–3 on the scale then that's great.

The theory is that 70% of your maximum heartrate or the Maffetone Method heartrate (180 minus your age) should correlate with 4–5 on the RPE scale.

If you find that you're at 7–9 on the scale, then slow down a bit or just give yourself a very short interval and see how you feel and recover. It's harder to recover from high intensity exercise, and you can only sustain that for short periods of time.

You can track your exercise heartrate or RPE scores in your journal or a spreadsheet.

Recovery heartrate – RecHR

How quickly your heartrate comes down after exercise is a good indication of recovery, physical wellbeing, your ability to tolerate exercise and increased fitness.

This is particularly important during and after cancer treatment, as it can help structure how much exercise you can do, and how much intensity you can manage. It can also be an indication of excess fatigue or other illness.

If your heartrate stays high for a while after exercise, it's a sign you're struggling to recover, you're very fatigued or your medication is affecting your ability to tolerate much exercise.

How to measure your RecHR

Using your watch or monitor, at the end of your exercise session, watch how long it takes for your heartrate to drop. The faster the better.

Make a note of the number (bpm) at 1 minute and 5 minutes after stopping exercise.

Example:

Before exercise –	heartrate = 65 bpm
During exercise –	heartrate = 135 bpm
1 minute post exercise –	heartrate = 110 bpm
5 minutes post exercise –	heartrate = 70 bpm

This would indicate a good recovery and someone who is fit and responsive to exercise. At 5 minutes post exercise, their heartrate is pretty much back to the pre-exercise rate. All you need to do is monitor your recovery heartrate at 1 minute and 5 minutes and notice how it responds.

As I've said, if you find it takes a long time to drop after exercise, this could indicate that you're fatigued or exercising too hard. Next time lower the intensity or shorten the duration of your exercise. If it's still high (>120 bpm) 5 minutes after exercise, then consult your doctor.

I use heartrate training with all my clients, not just those with cancer. And it's a great way to make sure you're getting the most out of your exercise, not working too hard and it gives you some parameters to structure your exercise sessions.

Using heartrate to monitor the effectiveness of your exercise routine doesn't have to be difficult. Here's a quick summary.

1.   There are three heartrate numbers to know: your RESTING rate (RHR), your

EXERCISE rate (EHR) and your RECOVERY rate (RecHR).

2. Monitor your RESTING heartrate (RHR) and know your average. If it's getting lower over time, this is a sign of increased fitness. Use an app (see page 198) to measure something called heartrate variability in order to give you more insight into your recovery/stress load on the body.

3. If your RESTING heartrate is 5–10 beats higher than normal, then it's a sign of fatigue, stress, lack of recovery or illness. It's best to rest that day. If it's much higher than normal (20–30 beats), then see your doctor or call your oncology team.

4. Calculate your EXERCISE heartrate (EHR) using the Maffetone Method (180 minus your age) or use a rating of perceived exertion (RPE) of around 5/10 effort level for the majority of your exercise sessions. This helps you get the most out of your exercise without working too hard.

5. Monitor your RECOVERY heartrate (RecHR) after exercise to see how well you're tolerating exercise and to structure your next session. The faster it drops the fitter you are and the better you are able to tolerate exercise.

6. An unusually elevated heartrate any time BEFORE, DURING or AFTER exercise can be a cause for concern, so do speak to your doctor if it stays high or there is an unusual response.

7. It doesn't have to be complicated. Heartrate training is a really smart and simple way to make sure you don't overdo it and you get the most out of your exercise.

Key points

- Remember that 'fitness' is individual – being 'fit' is relative to you as a person, but also where you are in relation to your cancer journey and treatment. You might need to rethink what 'fitness' means to you, especially if you were very fit before diagnosis. Just getting out of bed and around the block for a walk can be a huge achievement some days and should be celebrated. So, keep it in perspective and be kind to yourself.

- Take things back to basics. Wipe the slate clean and draw a line in the sand, especially if you were super fit before cancer. You are where you are right now. Don't compare yourself to the past or hope for more in the future – just accept where you are right now in this moment. Regular exercisers are likely to find it hard to go back to being a 'beginner' again, but that's what you must do; don't beat yourself up about it.

- Keep in mind the six components of 'fitness' and how they interconnect – strength, balance, flexibility, cardiovascular fitness, body composition and co-ordination/ agility. Each component is important in its own right, but so is how they connect with each other. Identify any components you feel need work and focus your efforts there or choose activities that help develop them, especially during treatment when muscle loss is more likely. Tai Chi for balance, or jogging/walking for cardiovascular fitness for example, or strength training for muscle loss.

- Keep the FITT principles in mind – frequency, intensity, type and time – when planning any activities to help ensure you don't do too much too soon, but also to help you get the intensity and dose right. Only increase one principle at a time and work on 'frequency' first. Consistency is the goal, although remember every day will be different and you might not be able to plan ahead too far.

- If you were very active prior to diagnosis, you might need to reduce time/intensity of an activity by as much as 50–75% (or even more) until you know how much your body can tolerate and recover from. What you can do during cancer treatment is likely to be very different from what you could regularly do before diagnosis.

- Your resting heartrate (RHR) can tell you a lot about your body, fitness and health. Measure it first thing in the morning either manually by counting your pulse or with an app on your phone or a watch with a sensor. Your RHR will help you monitor the stress load on your body and your improving fitness (the lower it goes the fitter you're getting), but an unusual reading can also help you identify any illnesses or signs of additional stress on your body. During cancer treatment and afterwards it's a useful tool to reduce overtraining risk.

- Monitoring your exercise heartrate (EHR) is a smart way to keep the intensity of your exercise on track. Calculate what your 'working rate' should be and stick to it religiously. It helps you tune into your body and provides structure, so you don't do too much or too little. It can also highlight improvements in fitness (as you get fitter it'll be lower for the same effort) or be used to flag up any problems if you notice an especially high heartrate.

- Also remember that during and after cancer treatment there is no linear progression to recovery and exercise ability. Every day will be different. Some days you'll feel great, on others you may not be able to get out of bed. A bad day doesn't mean you've gone backwards, it just means you're having a bad day. Tune into your body and go with the flow. Learn to be flexible and respond to how you're feeling. Learn when to push yourself a bit, and equally, when you really do need to take it easy and rest.

Chapter 7

Core exercises and rehabilitation after surgery

The majority of people with colorectal cancer will have surgery. There are many different types of surgery depending on the size and location of the tumour and your health, age, physical wellbeing and fitness. Some people might have multiple extensive surgeries and other people may only have one keyhole procedure. Many patients are also given a stoma. In all cases, abdominal surgery is a major procedure and not to be underestimated.

You should get lots of support from your surgeon, the nurses and physiotherapists and in time you will recover and get better, but it can feel like quite a shock, both physically and mentally. Initially after surgery you might feel like you can't stand up straight, and even walking might feel difficult. It's common to protect your stomach, to develop a hunched posture and feel frail, weak and a bit like you've been hit by a truck. It's hard to imagine ever being able to lift anything ever again or get back to basic activities, let alone back to doing any sport or fitness. But in time you will. Your body simply needs time to heal, repair and get stronger.

How long does it take to recover from surgery?

How long it takes to recover from surgery is different for everyone and dependent on many factors. The type of surgery you had and how extensive it was (laparoscopic/laparotomy, stoma formation and reconstruction of the pelvic floor) and if you had any complications; how poorly you were before; other treatments; your age/fitness and general health all play a part in how quickly you will recover.

Generally, it's considered that six weeks is the average time for someone to be back to 'normal' activities, back to work and able to engage in exercise and to be 'recovered' after major abdominal surgery. The six-week timeline seems to be fairly standard advice after all types of surgery (even after childbirth or a Caesarean) and is roughly based on tissue healing time – in that it takes six weeks for your tissues to fully heal.

However, it's not a 'one size fits all' timeline. If you're having chemo, radiotherapy or have had more major surgery or complications, things will be different and you may take much longer or have more than one 'recovery cycle'. And likewise, if you're otherwise healthy and fit, and had a relatively uncomplicated operation, you may find you bounce back much faster than six weeks. And that's fine too.

Don't compare yourself with anyone else. Your recovery timeline is yours and yours alone. Don't be rushed to do too much too soon. But equally, if you feel well and want to do more, then don't feel held back or restricted. So much of recovery is about rebuilding confidence. The more you can move and get your muscles working for you again, the more confident you'll feel.

Much of your recovery is down to you. There's loads you can do to help yourself, get stronger sooner and rebuild your confidence faster. Here are some top tips.

1. Try to avoid being too sedentary and inactive – just aim to move a bit more.
2. Get up, get out and get some fresh air – go for a walk every day.
3. Do some core exercises to strengthen your muscles and rebuild your confidence (see page 103).
4. Focus on good hydration and nutrition (see Chapter 9) to help your body heal. Include fruit and vegetables and lots of protein-rich foods for healing.
5. Get enough rest and sleep – your body is using up a lot of energy to heal itself – but get the right balance.

The table on page 94 gives a potential timeline for an 'active recovery'. Bear in mind this is just a rough guide, and everyone will be different. However, this timeline gives you some structure for what you *might* be able to expect after an uncomplicated laparoscopic bowel resection and/or stoma formation, if you were fit and otherwise well prior to surgery.

Days post-operation	Activity
First 7–10 days	3–4 days post-surgery – commence gentle core, breathing and pelvic floor exercises 2–3 x per day Discharged from hospital approx. 3–5 days Walking – twice daily 10 minutes (more if tolerated)
10–14 days	Continue with core, breathing and pelvic floor exercises 2–3 x per day Walking – increase to 20 minutes x 2 per day
Week 3–4	Progress to more advanced core exercises (see Chapter 8) and include general conditioning exercises for strength, flexibility and mobility Progress walking further – build up to 40–60 minutes per day if possible; start to walk more briskly
Week 5–6	Continue with core exercises (from Chapter 8) and daily walking Gradual return to normal daily activities – gentle housework, work and light gardening A gentle/progressive return to swimming, Pilates, gym workouts or jogging if desired. Keep sessions short and monitor recovery rate Avoid heavy and awkward lifting. Lift with good technique
Week 6–12	Gradual return to more active sports, competition and normal activities Continue with core/pelvic floor and breathing exercises forever!

Core restoration

From a rehabilitation perspective, everyone who has had any kind of abdominal surgery (anything below the chest) should be advised to do some specific rehabilitation exercises after their operation. Specific gentle exercises are important to regain function and strength in your core/pelvic muscles and to rebuild your confidence.

One common theme that patients describe after bowel surgery is the sense of losing control of their stomach muscles and feeling they have no 'core strength'. This can have a knock-on effect to balance, co-ordination, back, hip and knee pain and generally feeling lacking in confidence and fear of moving, even doing basic daily activities. Many people complain of backache in the post op period and this change in core function (see page 96) is one of the reasons.

What do patients say?

Here are a few comments from patients who have had bowel surgery, and their thoughts on the 'core rehabilitation process':

'We should be cared for by a physio to begin to work out an individual exercise routine. We need to know what we CAN do'

'I'd love to know "dos and don'ts" of exercise'

'There's a need for more advice about abdominal exercises'

'More information is needed in this area about abdominal exercises'

'Try to go out every day, even if it's just for 10 mins around the block'

'We are vulnerable after surgery. Should not have to do chasing information. People don't know what to ask for'

'I have tried to strengthen my core and now feel pretty strong 5 months after surgery'

'Too often patients are not advised of the dos and don'ts after surgery. Physical rehabilitation after surgery should be standard practice'

'Exercise is so important in the recovery process. But it's never discussed'

'I wish I'd known what I could and couldn't do'.

These comments prove the need for the exercises in this chapter. I hope that now you've found this book, you'll get the advice you need and feel more confident.

Here's a quick question if you've already had abdominal surgery.
*   How confident do you feel about doing core exercises?

1	2	3	4	5	6	7	8	9	10
Not at all confident									Extremely confident

Score yourself on the scale and we'll come back to it later.

Your 'core'

Your 'core' is vital and plays a part in every movement you do. As you'll know, simple things like getting in and out of bed can become surprisingly difficult after surgery. You suddenly realise that you use your core muscles all the time for every movement you make.

A rehabilitation programme of exercises to gently strengthen these muscles after surgery is vitally important. When damaged (through surgery) the muscles 'switch off' and your entire core function changes. Gentle rehab exercises will help you to 'reconnect' with your deep core muscles and start to restore normal function. Tiny gentle movements can make a huge difference. I like to think of it as a 'springboard' to getting moving again and back to daily life. It's about putting the foundations back in place and rebuilding strength and connection with the muscles.

But there are two main problems we see in getting patients moving after surgery.

1.   Very few clinicians provide specific advice to patients after surgery, and the post-op instructions tend to be 'rest' or 'wait six weeks' or 'don't lift anything heavy'. This advice is unnecessarily cautious, restrictive and disabling. Patients are left feeling scared to move and if they 'rest completely' as per instructions, risk deconditioning (and losing confidence) even more. Then there is a spiral of fear, inactivity and less and less confidence, further muscle loss and further inactivity.

2.   And then we have the opposite problem. Patients (particularly those who were fit before) who do want to do 'core exercises' will often search on the internet and come up with 'classic' core exercises, such as planks, sit-ups and other challenging moves, which won't be appropriate in the post-op period. These exercises are 'fitness training' exercises and too challenging in the early days.

What we need to do is restorative rehabilitation moves instead. They are very different. So instead, there needs to be a step-by-step programme of restorative movements, rehabilitation and progressive exercises which take you through the first 6–12 weeks of recovery. This is about regaining control, connection, function and synergy in your core muscles, in a deep and intuitive way. And this is vital for EVERYONE.

Guidelines

The Association of Stoma Care Nurses (ASCN) guidelines[1] state that you can start gentle core exercises within 3–4 days after your surgery. If you feel well enough and not too sore, there's no reason why you can't start sooner.

However, that might be too soon for you, so start when you feel ready, even if it's weeks after your operation. Everyone is different and it's never too late. This advice is the same whether you had a full open procedure (laparotomy) or keyhole (laparoscopic), and applies to everyone who's had abdominal surgery, including those with a stoma. I believe that core exercises for bowel cancer patients should be embedded into care after surgery, much like exercise is for knee and hip replacement.

In the first few weeks after surgery, there are four things to focus on, and I will address each in turn in the following sections:

- pelvic floor exercises
- breathing techniques
- core/abdominal muscles
- walking.

Pelvic floor exercises

Anyone who has had bowel surgery should do pelvic floor exercises, especially if you are planning to have a stoma reversal (but check with your clinical team first – see box). Why? The pelvic floor is a vital, yet invisible, group of muscles and ligaments which form a sling deep at the bottom of your pelvis (see Figure 7.1), holding your pelvic organs (bowel, bladder, uterus etc) in place and controls your continence and sexual function.

It's vital for everyone to have a strong and well-functioning pelvic floor, regardless of whether you're 80 or 18, male or female, or whether you've had surgery or not. The pelvic floor works in synergy with the other muscles of the 'core' – abdominal wall, back muscles and diaphragm – and is a REALLY important muscle group that often gets neglected.

Check first

If you've had extensive pelvic or rectal surgery or the cancer has spread into the pelvic floor muscles, then please check with your surgeon or nurse before you start pelvic floor exercises. If you're already seeing an incontinence/bowel specialist, please speak to them and follow their advice about the exercises in this book.

Some surgeries involve removal of some of the pelvic floor muscle and reconstruction using other muscles in the body. That situation is beyond the scope of this book, so please speak with a specialist physiotherapist. You will need to do rehab exercises for your pelvic floor but may need slightly different advice or support.

In people who have had their rectum removed (a procedure known as a panproctocolectomy), you can and should do pelvic floor exercises. They may also help with healing and pain management. But start gently with a few gentle 'squeezes' first and see how you feel.

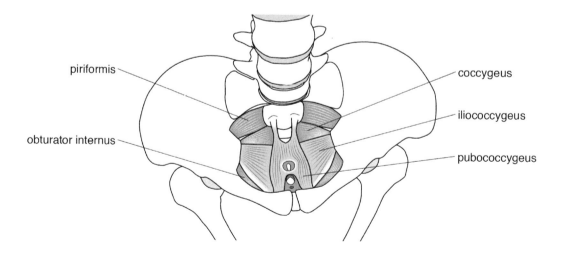

Figure 7.1 The pelvic floor

Most people simply don't do pelvic floor exercises often enough, so they end up not being effective. You do need to do a 'set' of exercises three times per day, every day, for best results. But they really don't need to be hard or complicated. Try to integrate them into your life, so you do them in the car, when watching TV, when in a meeting at work, sitting reading with the kids, even when cooking or washing up.

Tip: find a cue – maybe when you're waiting for the kettle to boil or when talking on the phone – and get into the habit of always doing a set then. See page 198 for details of a useful resource, the 'NHS Squeezy' App, to help you remember. The pelvic floor is an internal muscle. When you are doing your squeezes, no-one should be able to tell from the outside of your body. It's a 'secret' exercise.

How to do pelvic floor exercises

Start gently. If you've just had surgery in the last few days or weeks, start with VERY gentle and VERY short (1–2 seconds) squeezes and see how you respond. Build up slowly and gently.

You need to do two types of exercise to work the muscles in different ways – long squeezes and quick flicks.

Long squeeze

You might want to get someone to read the following instructions out to you, so you can concentrate and do the exercise with your eyes closed.

1. Sit on chair with your feet flat on the floor. Sit upright with good posture. Imagine a balloon pulling the crown of your head to the ceiling. OR
2. Lie on your back with your knees bent, keeping everything relaxed. This is an easier position if you've just had surgery or you struggle to 'find' the muscles.
3. Relax your whole body and the muscles of your legs, buttocks and upper body. Breathe in and out a few times and make sure your pelvic floor is relaxed.
4. Then take a gentle inhale, and as you EXHALE gently tighten your back passage as if you're trying to prevent breaking wind. Then, continue to squeeze, and tighten your front passage as if you're trying to stop the flow of urine. It's a feeling of pulling up inside. Do not tense any other muscles in your legs or bottom. You should feel like you're pulling the sling of muscle up inside, as if your sit bones are being drawn together. (For men: a good cue is to get the sensation that you're pulling your testicles up inside your body.)

5. Hold the squeeze for 3–5 seconds to begin with, building up to 10 seconds maximum. Keep breathing gently!
6. You might find this hard, so even if you just manage 1 second to begin with, that's fine. Build on that and work up to 3–5 seconds and then more.
7. Then relax for 10 seconds. Allow the pelvic floor to gently drop and relax away completely.
8. Repeat and relax again.
9. Remember to breathe throughout.
10. Repeat this 5–10 times. If you feel you're starting to fatigue, then rest for a while and try again later.

Quick flicks

These work the 'fast twitch' muscle fibres and are a little more challenging. 'Quick flicks' are where you pull the pelvic floor up fast, then relax it.

1. Count quickly 'one and two and three and four and five and six and seven and eight and nine and ten' pulling your pelvic floor up on the number 'count'.
2. Do a set of 10 quick flicks.
3. Relax for a few minutes. Then repeat.

Do one set of 10 long holds and two sets of 10 quick flicks three times per day.

If you're finding it hard to 'locate' the muscle or you're not sure if you're doing the exercise properly, or you feel 'bulging' rather than pulling up, then ask your GP to refer to you a bowel/continence or women's health physiotherapist or see a specialist nurse.

Breathing techniques

Breathing has a huge impact on our physical health, mental wellbeing and core control. Most of us don't breathe properly or deeply enough. The diaphragm is an internal muscle and is part of the 'core'. It works in synergy with the other muscles of the core – the pelvic floor, abdominal wall and back muscles. Breathing is essentially a core exercise. Imagine your core like a 'can' with a top (your diaphragm) and a bottom (your pelvic floor). After surgery, we tend to take shallow breaths, which can affect the way the core muscles work. This can become a habit and can result in poor core function in the long term.

There are two different types of breathing exercise I want you to try here. One is to encourage deep breathing and is good for relaxation/pain (and prevention of complications after surgery).

The other is more active 'umbrella' breathing and is to encourage your core muscles to work efficiently. There are slight variations between the two techniques but give both a try.

Deep breathing for relaxation

When you have had surgery or are anxious, fatigued or in pain, your breathing tends to become shallow and faster, your heartrate can rise, and your blood pressure can increase. This is the 'fight or flight' response to stress.

Deep breathing can help relax you and reduces feelings of anxiety. It helps to regulate your nervous system and calms the stressful 'fight or flight' response. Using your breath correctly can help bring calm to your body, slow your heartrate and encourage you to breathe more deeply, taking more oxygen into your body. It's really simple to do but needs some concentration.

Note: '2 to 4 breathing' means breathing in for 2 seconds and out for 4.

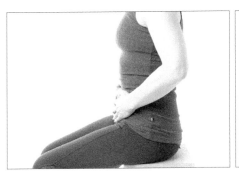 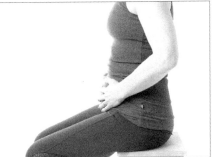

Let's try it.
- Sit relaxed on a chair or stool (as in the figure above) or propped up in bed. Place your hands on your lower belly.
- Close your eyes. Breathe in through your nose for a count of 2 seconds, then exhale slowly (again through your nose) for a count of 4. So, your breath out is twice as long as your breath in.
- Allow your breath to gently rise and fall.

- Feel your belly softly expand into your hands when you inhale (see the Figure on page 101). Feel the breath move deeply into your abdomen, not just the upper part of your chest.
- Try a count of 2–4 to begin with and increase it to breathing in for 3 and out for 6, or breathing in for 8 and out for10 as you get more proficient. Breathe in and out gently through your nose without forcing it.
- Try this for 1–2 minutes initially and experiment with the ratios, body position and length of practice. Try doing it when you feel anxious and/or throughout the day.

'Umbrella' breathing for core and diaphragm activation

This type of breathing exercise helps to engage your core muscles and teaches you how to expand your ribs correctly. It's a little more 'active', so if you've just had surgery then go gently to start with.

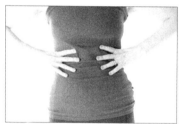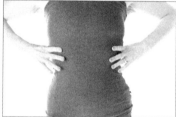

Let's try it.
- Sit upright on a chair or the side of your bed, or stand tall. Wrap your hands around your lower ribs, with fingers at the front and thumbs at the back. Relax your shoulders.
- Breathe in deeply through your nose and aim to fill your hands with your ribs – keeping your shoulders down. Let your ribs expand out to the sides and feel your hands move away as they open up (see Figure above) – like an umbrella. Your abdomen will inflate a little, but not too much. Feel the breath in your ribs mostly.
- Then exhale slowly through your mouth and actively bring your ribs down using your abdominal muscles. You should feel your ribs move clearly away from your hands, as though you're trying to close an umbrella. Be sure not to inflate your abdomen at all as you breathe out. In fact it should feel as if it is flattening.
- Relax and repeat 5 or 6 times.

> **Note**
> If you have a more complex breathing issue (such as COPD) or have lung cancer, then ask to speak to a respiratory physiotherapist who can help you with specific advice.

Core abdominal exercises

Your 'core' is technically a group of four muscles, not just your abdominal wall as many people mistakenly think. Imagine the 'core' as a canister with two walls, a top and bottom (see Figure 7.6).

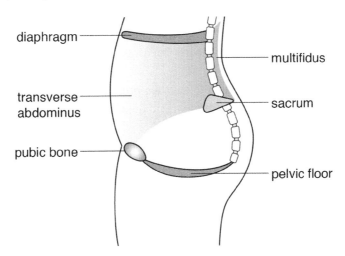

Figure 7.6 The core muscles

The core comprises:
* the pelvic floor
* the abdominal wall
* the back muscles
* the diaphragm – hence why breathing is so important.

I'd argue that the core extends even further and includes shoulder muscles, glutes (buttock muscles), low back and hip muscles. However, let's stay focused on the 'core canister' for now to keep things simple.

103

Your core muscles provide spinal stability and are essential in maintaining posture, continence and protecting your organs. In other words, we need them to be working well for us for the rest of our lives. Signs that your core isn't working well for you include incontinence, pelvic prolapse, hernia, breathing difficulties and all sorts of back, hip and musculoskeletal issues. Even the knees and feet can be affected if the core isn't working effectively.

If you have had surgery anywhere in your abdominal wall or pelvic floor, your muscles will be weakened and compromised. The first step is regaining control, connection and synergy in the core as a whole.

Core 1 *Core restoration programme*

This programme of nine exercises is the foundation for everyone, even if you're fit and healthy or your cancer treatment has been relatively straightforward. Don't be tempted to skip it.

In most cases you should be able to start the programme within 3–4 days of your surgery, even if you have a long central wound or stoma. Progress gently through the exercises and listen to your body.

Note

Some low-grade discomfort after surgery is normal and to be expected. So, don't wait until you're completely pain free. You may find gentle movements will help, as they improve blood flow and circulation and can aid healing (and pain). But do go gently. If you experience severe or sharp pains or the movements make pain worse, then back off and make the movement easier or try something different.

You can also do these movements any time before or after surgery.

Before surgery

If you're reading this BEFORE you have surgery, then brilliant! Get started now and practise all the moves, so you know what you're doing after your operation. The fitter and stronger you are BEFORE your surgery the better. This is something called 'pre-habilitation' and various research studies have shown that people who do exercise

BEFORE their surgery or treatment have better outcomes (see Chapter 2).

Waiting for surgery can be an anxious time but focusing on some exercises which will help you in the long term can be really beneficial, giving you a sense of control and positivity.

Post-surgery – months or years

If you're reading this and your surgery was months or even years ago, it's never too late to start. If you've never done rehabilitation exercises, it's likely your core won't be functioning well, so start with this programme and follow the exercises in order. You will progress more quickly but start here.

Important – All of these movements should be done slowly with control. Don't rush through them. Focus and concentrate and do them with precision and the best technique you can manage.

Exercise 1 Deep core control

When can you start it?	Where can you do it?
3–4 days post-surgery	In bed or on the floor

This is the starting point for everyone. This exercise teaches you to 'reconnect' with your deep abdominal muscles – the TVA or transverse abdominis (see Figure 7.7). The TVA works in synergy with the pelvic floor, so you must get both working together. You need to be able to activate and connect with this muscle, before you can continue to strengthen it.

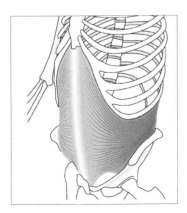

Figure 7.7 The transverse abdominal muscle or TVA

This is another 'internal' exercise, so no-one should know you're doing it. Nothing moves on the outside. It's a feeling of pulling your low/deep abdominal muscles in and towards your spine.

You can do this exercise when standing, sitting or lying on your back or side – instructions for each are given below. It can be tricky to feel initially but keep trying and you'll get there. Start by lying on your back (see Figure 7.8) and then follow the instructions below. Ask someone to read them out to you.

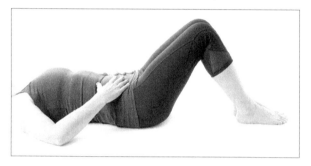

Figure 7.8 Deep core – back

- Lie on your back (on your bed or on the floor) with knees bent. Relax completely.
- Rest your hands on your lower abdomen – so you can feel the muscles working when you do the exercise. You can feel the muscles if you press your fingers into your abdomen 5 cm (2 in) in from your hip bones. You should feel a tightening under your fingers. Relax everything.
- Then take a deep breath in through your nose. As you exhale through your mouth, imagine pulling your ribs down towards your pelvis and gently draw your abdominal muscles inwards and towards your spine. Imagine you're pulling your hip bones together like two covers of a book. See if you can feel the muscles in your deep abdomen – you're looking for a feeling of tension under your fingers.
- Nothing moves on the outside of your body.
- Hold this contraction for 2–3 seconds – keep breathing – and release.
- Repeat 5 times.
- Build up to holding the contraction for 10 seconds and repeat 5–10 times.

You can also do this lying on your side – see Figure 7.9 on the opposite page – and follow the instructions that follow it. This might be easier initially if you're struggling to do the exercise lying on your back.

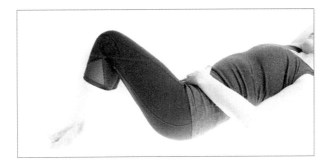

Figure 7.9 Deep core – side

- Lie on your side (on your bed or on the floor) with knees bent.
- Rest your hand on your lower abdomen – so you can feel the muscles working.
- Allow your stomach to drop into your hand toward the floor – and be completely relaxed.
- Then take a deep breath in. As you exhale, pull your ribs down towards your pelvis and gently draw your abdominal muscles inwards and towards your back. You should feel your belly lift up away from your hand.
- Nothing moves on the outside of your body.
- Hold this contraction for 2–3 seconds and release.
- Repeat 5 times.

You can also try this exercise sitting down (as in Figures 7.10 and 7.11). When you get practised at it, you can do it when watching TV, in the car, on the train, when sat at work or in the cinema!

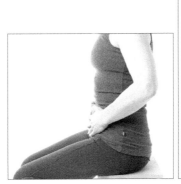
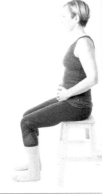

Figure 7.10 and 7.11 Deep core – seated Notice how the belly pulls in, away from the hands

Exercise 2 Pelvic tilt

When can you start it?	Where can you do it?
3–4 days post-surgery	In bed or on the floor

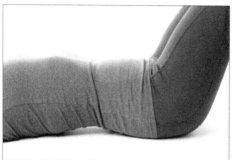 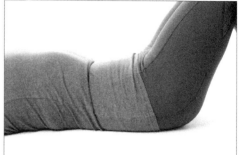

Figure 7.12 (a) and (b) Pelvic tilt

- Lie on your back, knees bent and completely relax.
- Imagine you have a small ball resting on your stomach – half way between your navel and your pubic bone.
- Inhale through your nose, then as you exhale tilt your pelvis toward your face – as if you're rolling the ball into your navel.
- You'll get a feeling of your back gently flattening into the floor or your bed, but don't force it.
- Imagine trying to pull your ribs down and shorten the gap between the bottom rib and pelvis.
- Relax your legs and bottom and then hold the position for a second. Try not to push through your legs.
- Return to neutral position and relax.
- Inhale again, then exhale and repeat.
- Repeat gently 5–10 times.
- As you get stronger, contract your abdominal muscles deeply at the same time you rock back with your pelvis.

Exercise 3 Knee rolls

When can you start it?	Where can you do it?
3–4 days post-surgery	In bed or on the floor

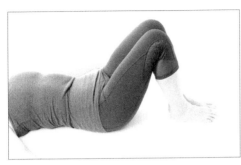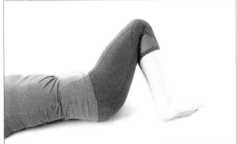

Figure 7.13 (a) and (b) Knee rolls

- Lie on your back, with knees bent, and relax.
- Keep your knees together.
- Gently let your knees roll over to one side – only go a small way to begin with.
- Return to centre and repeat on the other side. Don't allow your opposite shoulder to lift.
- Do this with perfect and slow control, using your abdominal muscles to draw your legs back to centre.
- Repeat 10–15 times. Keep breathing gently throughout.
- As you get stronger, let your knees drop further across and contract your abdominal muscles more strongly to pull them back over.

Exercise 4 Seated knee lifts

When can you start it?	Where can you do it?
3–4 days post-surgery	In bed or on the floor

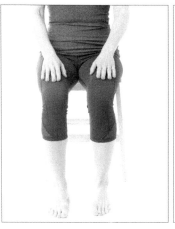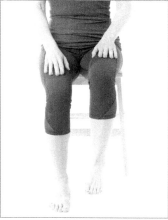

Figure 7.14 (a) Neutral position and (b) Seated knee lift

- Sit tall on a chair with your back unsupported away from the back of the chair.
- Engage your deep abdominal muscles and continue to breathe.
- Stabilise your core and then slowly lift one foot from the floor – about 2 cm.
- Replace your foot and switch to the other side. Make sure your torso doesn't rock from side to side.
- Repeat this 10–20 times slowly and with control. Keep your abdominal muscles engaged throughout and keep breathing.

Exercise 5 Tilt on hands and knees

When can you start it?	Where can you do it?
7–10 days post-surgery	Ideally on the floor

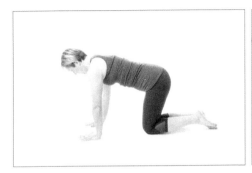 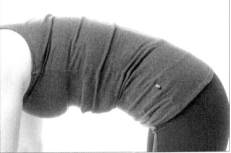

Figure 7.15 (a) and (b) Tilt on hands and knees

- On your hands and knees on all fours. Pop a cushion under your knees if you're not comfortable. Relax and breathe. Draw your stomach away from the floor and flatten your back. Relax through your shoulders and neck.
- Inhale through your nose, then as you exhale, gently tuck your pelvis under, curling your tailbone under, keeping your head and upper body still.
- Imagine you have a headlight on your pubic bone! Try to shine the light up along the floor and onto the wall in front of you.
- Return back to a neutral/flat back position and repeat.
- Repeat 10 times.
- As you get stronger, try to engage more of your abdominal muscles as you curl under.
- If you can't get onto all fours, you can do this move standing next to a desk or kitchen worktop for support.

Exercise 6 Knee drops

When can you start it?	Where can you do it?
7–10 days post-surgery	Ideally on the floor but can be done in bed

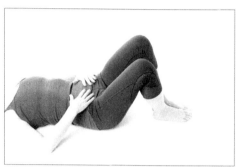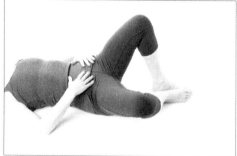

Figure 7.16 (a) and (b) Knee drops

- Lie on your back, with knees bent, and relax.
- Tighten your deep abdominal muscles – as in the Exercise 1 and create a small pelvic tilt.
- Breathe and relax – but keep the deep engagement in your core.
- Slowly allow one knee to drop away towards the floor/bed while maintaining control of your pelvis.
- Bring the knee back to centre and repeat on the other side.
- Imagine you have a glass of champagne balancing on your knee and keep your knee very still as the opposite knee drops away.
- Keep control of your core the entire time, so no rocking or rolling. Do this very slowly.
- Only go down as low as you feel comfortable. The goal is not to try and get your knee to the floor.
- Repeat 12–15 times.

Exercise 7 Heel lifts

When can you start it?	Where can you do it?
7–10 days post-surgery	Ideally on the floor but can be done in bed

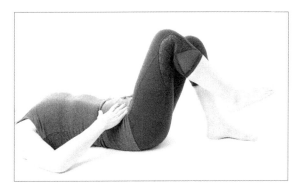

Figure 7.17 Heel lifts

- Lie on your back, with knees bent, and relax.
- Tighten your deep abdominal muscles – as in the Exercise 1.
- Breathe and relax – but keep the deep engagement in your core.
- Gently lift one foot off the floor/bed, maintaining control – only lift a small amount – no more than a few centimetres/inches.
- Replace your foot and repeat on the other side.
- Keep control of your core the entire time.
- Repeat 12–15 times.

Exercise 8 Leg slides

When can you start it?	Where can you do it?
7–10 days post surgery	Ideally on the floor but can be done in bed

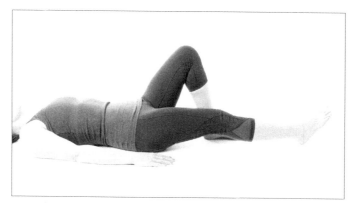

Figure 7.18 Leg slides

- Lie on your back, with knees bent, and relax.
- Tighten your deep abdominal muscles – as in Exercise 1.
- Breathe and relax – but keep the deep engagement in your core.
- Inhale through your mouth, then as you exhale gently slide one foot along the floor/bed, maintaining control of your pelvis, until your leg is straight.
- Pull your leg back in and repeat on the other side with the same breathing pattern. It's important to breathe OUT as you slide the leg away.
- Keep control of your core the entire time.
- Repeat 12–15 times.
- As you get stronger you can allow your heel to lift off the floor, straightening your leg parallel to the floor.

Exercise 9 Bridge

When can you start it?	Where can you do it?
7–10 days post surgery	Ideally on the floor but can be done in bed

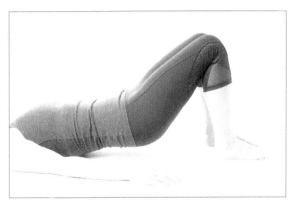

Figure 7.19 Bridge

- Lie on your back, with knees bent, and relax.
- Tighten your deep abdominal muscles – as in the first exercise.
- Breathe and relax – but keep the deep engagement in your core.
- Inhale through your nose, then as you exhale create a pelvic tilt rolling the imaginary ball into your navel.
- Then allow your bottom to lift and peel your spine off the floor into a low bridge. Don't force your hips too high so it feels uncomfortable. Push through your heels so you get some engagement into your hamstrings and bottom muscles.
- Pause at the top of the bridge. Inhale again, then as you exhale, SLOWLY roll back down, one vertebra at a time, and finally untuck your pelvis.
- Relax then repeat the whole process 5–10 times.
- As you get stronger, try to contract your abdominals even tighter throughout the movement.

How often and when to do all these exercises?

- Aim to do three exercises 3 times per day. Choose a mix of different exercises each time.
- You don't have to do them all at once. Little and often is best.
- Most people can start these moves 3–4 days after abdominal surgery, or certainly within the first week.
- Just start gently and build up slowly so you're doing around 10-15 repetitions of each exercise.
- If you experience soreness or discomfort afterwards, then just back off for a couple of days, reduce the number of repetitions and do them more gently, building back up slowly.
- An ideal time to do them is in bed in the morning, or in the evening in front of the TV. Apart from the seated knee lifts, they can all be done in bed or on the floor.

How confident are you feeling now?

Now you've had a go at those exercises, score yourself on the 'confidence scale' again.

- How confident do you feel about doing core exercises?

1 Not at all confident	2	3	4	5	6	7	8	9	10 Extremely confident

Look back at the number you scored at the start of this chapter and see how it compares. I'm hoping it's gone up and you're feeling loads more confident about core exercises.

Use a journal

Some people find it useful to keep a 'recovery journal' of what they do and how they're feeling. Use a notebook or spreadsheet. Something like the example on the next page would work well.

Say you aim to do three exercises 3 times per day. Just make a note of the ones you do and also how you feel. You could include information about how far you walk too and some notes on your progression, as shown in the example.

	Mon	Tues	Wed	Thurs	Fri	Sat	Sun
1	Knee lifts x 20 Leg slides x 20 Knee drops x 20						
2	Seated knee lifts x 20 Knee rolls x 20 Bridge x 10						
3	Knee lifts x 20 Leg slides x 20 Knee drops x 20						
Notes	Definitely getting stronger. Feel so much better than last week. Managing 20 of each exercise rather than 10.						
Walking	20 mins to Sam's house and back						

Walking

One of the best things you can do in the post-op period, or during chemo treatment, is to get out walking. Walk, walk and walk some more!

Walking improves blood flow around the body, prevents muscle wastage in your legs and helps maintain mobility, balance and general condition. And there's nothing like some fresh air to help with your recovery. And if you can walk more briskly – getting your heartrate up – you'll get cardiovascular benefits too.

If you have had surgery, the nurses and physios will have expected you to walk up and down the ward every day, and now you're home you need to continue and do the same.

Add your walks to your journal, as shown. As you get stronger, you'll soon be able to monitor real progress and start to feel much better.

Here are some top walking tips.

- Little and often is best. Aim for 10-minute walks to begin with. Even just a couple of laps around the block is fine. Or aim for the postbox/next lamp post, or whatever, and set yourself a little goal each day. The sense of achievement can be huge!
- Try to do two short walks per day. It might feel more like a 'shuffle' initially, but stick with it and you'll soon find it gets easier.
- Build up slowly over time so eventually you're doing 20–30 minutes each day.
- During chemotherapy, you may find some days are better than others. Try to maintain consistency and get out for a walk even if you don't feel much like it. If you feel really exhausted just try to walk around the garden or local park in order to get outside to breathe some fresh air.
- Although I'm not a huge fan of technology, step counters or apps can be useful in this situation and can be motivating and encouraging as you progress. See page 198 for details of the apps available that I have found useful.
- Don't try to aim for 10,000 steps per day, rather just look to see how you can increase your step count day by day. Start with 250–500 step increments and build up each day. So, if for example you walk 1500 steps, the next day aim for 2000.
- It sounds obvious, but wearing trainers or sports shoes will be more comfortable, provide better grip and help you walk faster and more safely than standard shoes. Even though you might just be going round the block, there's something about lacing up trainers that makes it feel more purposeful and positive.
- Walk with good posture: head held high and chest lifted. Avoid slumping or holding your stomach. Walking with tall posture helps your core muscles engage and function better.
- Take a friend for company and support – arranging to meet a friend for a specific time will help you stick to a schedule.
- If you go out alone, take your phone.
- As you get stronger and fitter, try to walk more briskly so that your heartrate increases, and you get a little out of breath.
- The hardest part is getting out of the door. So, give yourself a little push even on days when you don't feel like it. Those are the days when you need it most.

Key points

- Post-op rehab exercises for your core muscles are a vital part of recovery for EVERYONE. Patients who do them often comment on how much better they feel – more positive and in control.
- Many people are surprised to learn they can start these exercises 3–4 days after surgery. This is a clinical guideline and recommendation from the Association of Stoma Care Nurses, but not every nurse or surgeon will be familiar with it. If they're not, ask them to read the *ASCN Clinical Guidelines*[1] or show them this book.
- Complete rest is not best for anyone. Most people are advised to go home and 'rest' for 6 weeks. This is not good advice, as people interpret it literally and sit on the sofa or rest in bed. This approach makes you feel like a 'patient' and increases fear-avoidance; also physically you're likely to decondition more. Instead, think about having an 'active recovery' balanced with gentle movement and appropriate rest. Try to be active every day during recovery. Short 10-minute walks and core exercises will really help rebuild your body and your mind.
- Walk, walk and walk some more. Walking is the best thing you can do in the post-op period.
- Everyone will recover differently and there is no 'one size fits all' solution. You have to listen to your body. Give it a little push from time to time, but equally rest if you feel you're doing too much.

Scan here to go directly to my website (www.theostomystudio.co.uk) where you will find videos and exercises.

Chapter 8

Advanced core and general fitness exercises

This chapter covers more advanced core exercises and a range of simple conditioning exercises you can do at home, as well as some modifications and adaptations to more vigorous exercises you might be used to doing for various sports.

However fit you used to be, please make sure you start with the 'Core 1 – Core restoration programme' (Chapter 7, page 104) first and that you feel comfortable with all those exercises before starting with the exercises in this chapter.

You might be ready to start this chapter within 2–4 weeks after your surgery, or a little later if you've had very extensive surgery or never done core exercises before.

First a quick recap on why this is so important.

1. To strengthen muscles that have been weakened directly through surgery – particularly the abdominal wall and core.
2. To rebuild confidence in your body and to reduce fear about moving and being active.
3. To recover faster and get back to day-to-day activities (lifting, shopping etc) and work.
4. To rebuild general strength throughout your whole body, especially after surgery and bed rest.
5. To create a 'foundation' for any future movement, especially for those who want to get back to sport, exercise and activity.
6. To reduce the risk of problems that might develop in the future – there's some evidence to show that strong core muscles may help to reduce your risk of developing a complication or hernia.

Kinesiophobia and body mistrust

Kinesiophobia is a term used to describe 'fear of movement'. When we experience pain, we become fearful of moving in the belief that it will make it worse. It's very common after surgery or an injury and can often lead to a spiral of immobility and increased pain in the long term, even though the body has healed. When we're sick, we also lose faith in our body and feel it's let us down – leading to a sense of body mistrust. Any movement might make things worse or cause pain. This is why it's so very important to start to get moving again after surgery and to re-build confidence in your body and in how you move. Any sort of rehabilitation and exercise programme can break this cycle of fear-avoidance and help to restore your confidence.

Core 2 Advanced core exercises

There are seven simple exercises here for you to try.
Knee circles
Bridge with ball/towel
Half Superman
Full Superman
Half dead bug
Full dead bug
Bridge with leg lift

If you're unsure how to do any of these exercises, please consult a qualified personal trainer (preferably one with training in postnatal rehab, as they tend to understand core rehabilitation best) or a cancer rehab/Pilates instructor or a physiotherapist.

Exercise 10 Knee circles

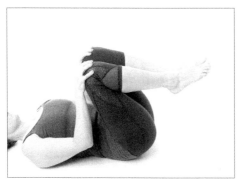 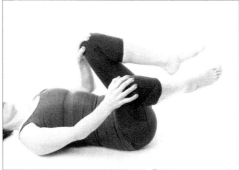

Figure 8.1 (a) and (b) Knee circles

- Lie on your back, with knees bent, and relax.
- Using your hands to lift your legs, bring your knees one at a time into your chest.
- Tighten your deep abdominal muscles – as described in the 'Deep core control' exercise in Chapter 7 (page 105).
- Place one hand on each knee.
- Make very slow circles with one knee, as if you're drawing a zero on the ceiling. Making them bigger makes the move more challenging.
- Repeat 10 times and then go in the opposite direction for 10.
- Repeat on the other side.
- Make the circles bigger to make it harder but maintain control of your abdominals and pelvis.

Exercise 11 Bridge with ball/towel

For this you'll need a rolled-up hand towel or a small, soft Pilates ball.

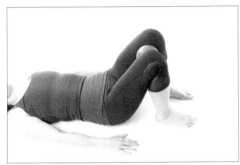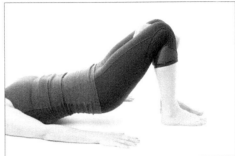

Figure 8.2 (a) and (b) Bridge with ball/towel

- Lie on your back, with knees bent, and relax.
- Place the ball or towel between your knees.
- Tighten your deep abdominal muscles. Breathe and relax – but keep the deep engagement in your core.
- Inhale through your nose, then exhale and gently tilt your pelvis towards your chest, rolling the ball into your navel as previously.
- Then allow your bottom to lift and peel your spine off the floor into a low bridge. Don't force your hips too high so it feels uncomfortable. Push through your heels so you get some engagement into your hamstrings and bottom muscles.
- At the same time, gently squeeze the ball/towel between your knees. Hold this position for a second or two.
- Pause at the top, then inhale and as you exhale, SLOWLY roll back down, one vertebra at a time, and finally untuck your pelvis.
- Relax then repeat the whole process 5–10 times.
- As you get stronger, try to contract your abdominals even tighter throughout the movement, squeeze the ball harder and hold the position for a count of 10.

Exercise 12 Half Superman

With arms

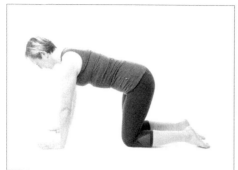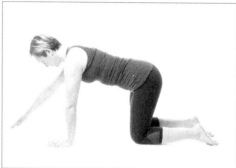

Figure 8.3 (a) and (b) Half Superman – with arms

- Start on your hands and knees. Make sure your hands are aligned under your shoulders and your hips are over your knees in a box position.
- Engage your deep abdominal muscles and control your trunk. Keep your shoulders strong and stable.
- Inhale, then as you exhale through your mouth, slowly slide the fingertips of one hand away from you keeping your arm straight. Do not move your knees or legs or allow your shoulders to drop.
- Slide your hand until your fingers just leave the floor, then pause and return your hand to the start position.
- Repeat on the other side. As you shift from side to side, aim to keep your shoulders very still.
- Maintain control of your core. Imagine you have a glass of water on your back and you need to balance so it doesn't fall off.
- Do 20 repetitions in total.

Exercise 12 Half Superman (cont'd)

With legs

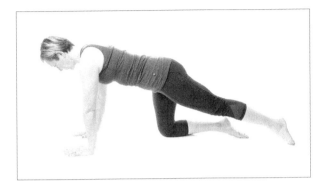

Figure 8.3 (c) Half Superman – with legs

- Start on your hands and knees. Make sure your hands are aligned under your shoulders and your hips are over your knees in a box position.
- Engage your deep abdominal muscles and control your trunk.
- Inhale. Then as you exhale, slowly slide your foot away, gradually straightening your leg.
- Slide your foot until your leg is straight, and your foot comes off the floor, pause and hold for a second. Then slowly slide it back.
- Repeat on the other side.
- Maintain control of your core. Imagine you have a glass of water on your back and you need to balance so it doesn't fall off.
- Do 20 repetitions in total.

Exercise 13 Full Superman

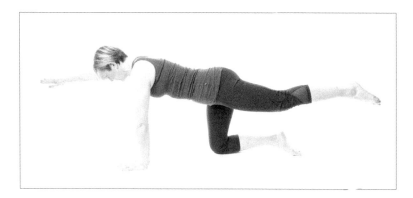

Figure 8.4 Full Superman

- Do this one when you've mastered the 'half Superman'. It puts both arms and legs together.
- Start on your hands and knees. Make sure your hands are aligned under your shoulders and your hips are over your knees in a box position.
- Engage your deep abdominal muscles and control your trunk.
- Inhale. The as you exhale, slowly straighten your left leg and opposite arm and slide until your hand and foot are both off the floor.
- Balance, pause and control your trunk – this is very important. Do not overextend your arm and leg. Control is the important thing here.
- Return your arm and leg to the start position with control.
- Repeat on the other side.
- Maintain control of your core. Imagine you have a glass of water on your back and you need to balance so it doesn't fall off.
- Do 20 repetitions in total.

Exercise 14 Half dead bug (optional – with balls)

If you want to do this exercise with weights, you can use Pilates balls (0.5 kg) or small hand weights that weigh around 0.5–1 kg. If you don't have any, use a can of food or a small water bottle in each hand.

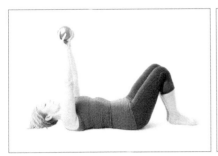 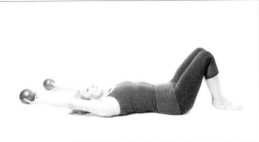

Figure 8.5 (a) and (b) Half dead bug

- Lie on your back, with knees bent.
- Hold your arms above your chest with arms straight – you can hold weights in your hands.
- Engage your deep abdominal muscles and breathe.
- Inhale. Then as you exhale (through your mouth), lower your arms over your head towards the floor – you can just do one arm at a time or both together.
- Keep your ribs pulled down and maintain control of your core. Exhaling helps to keep your ribs engaged.
- Return your arms to the start position and repeat.
- Do 20 repetitions in total.

Exercise 15 Full dead bug

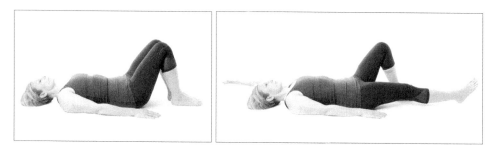

Figure 8.6 (a) and (b) Full dead bug

- Lie on your back, with knees bent.
- Engage your deep abdominal muscles and breathe.
- Inhale. Then as you exhale raise one arm over your head towards the floor – and at the same time extend the opposite leg until it's straight.
- Keep your ribs pulled down and maintain control of your core. Exhaling helps to keep your ribs engaged.
- Return to the start position and repeat.
- Do 10 repetitions in total.
- To make this a little more challenging, hold a small weight in each hand.

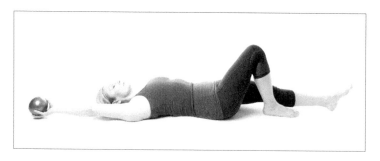

Figure 8.3 (c) Full dead bug with weights

Exercise 16 Bridge with leg lift

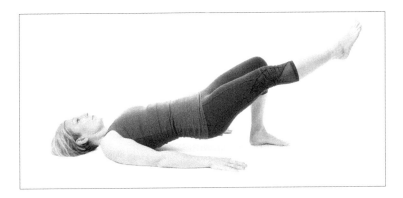

Figure 8.7 Bridge with leg lift

- Lie on your back, with knees bent, and relax.
- Tighten your deep abdominal muscles. Breathe and relax – but keep the deep engagement in your core.
- Inhale. Then as you exhale gently tilt your pelvis towards your chest, rolling the imaginary ball back into your navel as previously.
- Then allow your bottom to lift and peel your spine off the floor into a low bridge as in Figure 7.19 (page 115). Do not lift so high that it becomes uncomfortable.
- Slowly, with control, extend one leg so it's straight. Push through the heel on the floor so you get some engagement into your hamstrings and glute (buttock) muscles. Keep your pelvis level.
- Hold for 10–20 seconds.
- Return back to the bridge position then SLOWLY roll back down, one vertebra at a time, and finally untuck your pelvis.
- Relax then repeat the whole process 5–10 times on each side.

General fitness/conditioning exercises

There are 14 simple exercises in this section for you to try. You don't need to do them all. These exercises are for the whole body and are great for everyone. You can even do them at home in your slippers if you like!

They are a mixture of exercises to improve balance, flexibility, strength and core control – perfect if you've lost muscle through treatment or are just feeling a bit out of condition, or your muscles are generally tight or weak. They will help you manage everyday activities such as shopping, walking the dog, doing housework or just general lifting and moving – and also form the foundations if you want to become a bit more active or return to your chosen sport.

You don't need to do them all regularly, just try them all out at least once and see which ones you feel work best for you. They are designed to work on typical areas that people have problems with after surgery, bed rest or during treatment. Focus on the ones you feel you need most.

Design your own programme

But how do you know what's right for you? Below is a really simple exercise which may help you to identify areas of your body that need some TLC.

Mark on this body outline areas of concern – where you feel a bit stiff, tight, weak or sore. Then look at the exercises in this section and match them up with areas highlighted.

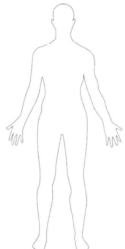

Area of concern	Choose these exercises
Weakness in your legs	Sit-stands (Exercise 23) and calf raises (Exercise 20)
Tightness in your thighs, possibly with knee pain	Foam rolling your quads (Exercise 29) and sit-stands (Exercise 23)
Weakness in your abdominal area	Core abdominal exercises (page 104)
Stiffness/soreness around your pelvis and buttocks	Massage ball in glutes (Exercise 30) and bridge with band (Exercise 26)

This is just an example. Go through the exercises yourself and think about what YOUR body needs, design your own programme and choose the right exercises for you.

Read through them, try them out and then create your own workout. Choose 3–4 movements to do each day and mix them up, repeating them several times during the day when you're on the phone, brushing your teeth, waiting for the kettle to boil and so on.

Area of concern	Choose these exercises

Use your journal or notebook to record which exercises you do and how you can progress them.

Exercise 17 Rotations

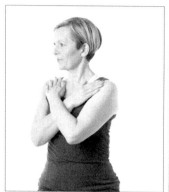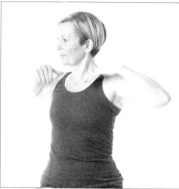

Figure 8.8 Rotations (a) Position 1; (b) Position 2

This exercise relieves tension in your mid upper back and is good if you've been in bed for a while or had abdominal surgery. Try this first thing in the morning on the side of your bed. Choose the position that is right for you.

Position 1

- Sit upright on a chair or the side of your bed.
- Cross your arms over your chest.
- Keep your hips fixed facing forward.
- With tall posture, rotate slowly to the right, then slowly to the left.
- Only go as far as you can – keep your shoulders down and keep breathing throughout.
- You should feel tension in your mid upper back.

Or

Position 2

- Place your fingers on your shoulders, with elbows out to the sides.
- Keep your hips fixed facing forward.
- With tall posture, rotate slowly to the right, then slowly to the left.
- Only go as far as you can – keep your shoulders down. Breathe out as you rotate and inhale as you return to the start position.
- You should feel tension in your mid upper back.

- Repeat 20–30 times slowly with control.

Exercise 18 Seated leg extension

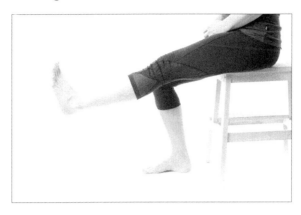

Figure 8.9 Seated leg extension

This exercise is good for strengthening the quadricep ('quads') muscles in your thighs.
- Sit upright in a chair or on the side of your bed.
- Slowly straighten one leg so you can feel your thigh muscle working, and pull your toes up towards you.
- Pause at the top, squeeze your thigh muscle, then return to the start position.
- Repeat this 10–20 times and then repeat on the other leg. Keep breathing naturally throughout.
- You can add a small 1 kg ankle weight if you desire.

Exercise 19 Standing glute squeeze

Get those super-important glute (bottom) muscles working after periods in bed or on the couch.

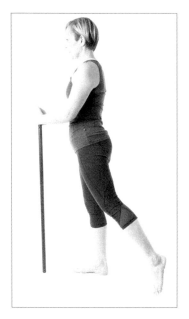

Figure 8.10 Standing glute squeeze

- Stand upright holding onto something for balance.
- Point your toe out behind you on a slight diagonal.
- Lift your toes about 5 cm (2 inches) from the floor; feel your bottom muscles working.
- Squeeze your glute muscle and pulse your leg with little lifts. Do not allow your back to arch. Keep your abdominals engaged and only lift with tiny movements.
- Make sure the hip on your 'standing' leg doesn't drop out to the side; keep it strong.
- Repeat 20 times and then repeat on the opposite leg.

Exercise 20 Calf raises

We lose muscle in the lower leg rapidly during/after treatment and bed rest. Rebuild calf strength with this exercise.

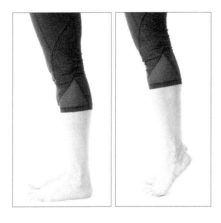

Figure 8.11 (a) Neutral position; (b) Calf raises

- Stand upright holding onto something in front of you (a chair or worktop) for balance.
- Slowly rise up onto the balls of your feet.
- Make sure you maintain tall posture and lift yourself 'up' rather than 'forward'.
- Keep your abdominal muscles engaged which stops you rocking forward. Imagine you're inside a tube and you're rising up and down inside.
- Lower yourself down and repeat 20 times 3 times per day.

NOTE – make sure your heels don't go out to the sides; push up through your big toes, NOT as shown in Figure 8.11(c).

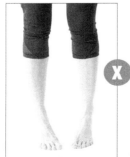

Figure 8.11 (c) Calf raises – avoid!

Exercise 21 Marching on the spot

This exercise is good for balance and leg strength, especially if you're feeling a bit frail.

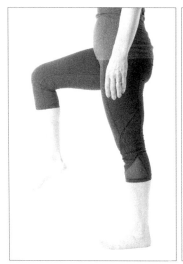 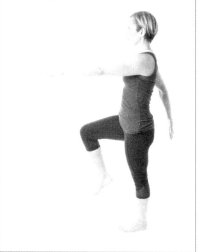

Figure 8.12 (a) Marching on the spot; (b) Marching on the spot with higher knees and arms swinging

- Stand upright holding onto something (a chair or worktop) to the side of you for balance.
- Slowly lift one foot, peeling it off the floor. Hold the position, then replace it and repeat on the other side, so you start to do a fluid marching movement.
- Work on good balance and hip control – avoid letting your hips sway from side to side and avoid any upper body movement from side to side.
- To make it harder, bring your knees higher and swing your arms.
- Repeat 20–30 marches 3 x per day.

Exercise 22 Clockface balance

This exercise is good for balance, co-ordination and leg strength. Start by holding on to something for balance until you are stronger and more balanced as in Fighre 8.13.

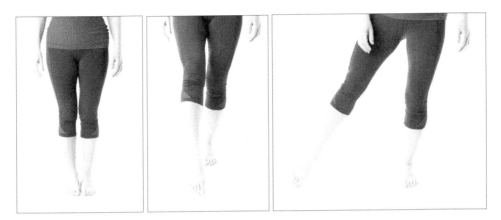

Figure 8.13 Clockface balance (a) Start position; (b) Toes point to 12 o'clock; (c) Toes point to 3 o'clock

- Stand upright holding onto something (a chair or worktop) to the side of you for balance.
- Balance on one leg and bend that knee slightly, maintaining tall posture.
- The idea of this exercise is to use your foot to point to imaginary positions on a clockface.
- Point to 12 on the clock (Figure 8.13 (b)), then 9 or 3, then 6 and return your foot to the start position Your standing leg should be doing the work.
- Repeat 5–6 times on each leg. Keep breathing throughout.
- As you get stronger and more balanced you can try this without holding onto anything.

Exercise 23 Sit-stand – variations

Leg strength is often lost during cancer treatment. Do these sit-stands every day to keep your legs strong. This is a super-simple exercise you can do at home at any time of the day. All you need is a chair. It's one of the most functional exercises and great for almost everyone.

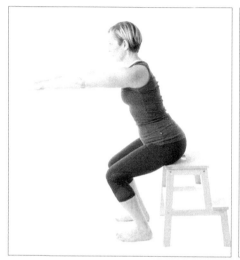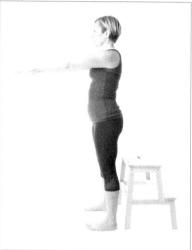

Figure 8.14 (a) and (b) Sit-stands with arms out infront

- Sit on a chair with either your arms folded OR out in front of you. If you're a bit unbalanced, make sure you have a support next to you.
- Have your feet at hip distance apart and firmly placed on the floor.
- Take a deep breath in, then use the power of your legs to push up to standing – exhaling as you come up. The exhalation is very important as this reduces pressure on your abdomen and pelvic floor.
- Pause, slowly lower yourself back down only briefly touching the chair rather than sitting, then push back up to standing again.
- Make sure your knees stay straight over your feet and don't drop inwards.
- If you're weak or just had surgery, sit and rest between each sit-stand and take your time.
- Initially just try 3–5 sit-stands 3 times per day.
- As you get stronger you can build up to 10–20 repetitions.

Exercise 24 Squats with balls

Pilates balls are optional; if you don't have them, do the exercise without, or use small water bottles or food cans instead.

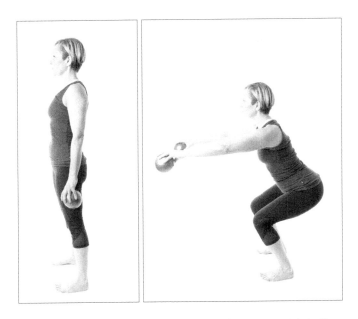

Figure 8.15 (a) Neutral position; (b) Squat with ball
– note, knees stay over toes

- Hold 0.5 kg Pilates balls or small weights in your hands.
- Stand upright holding the weights by your sides.
- Your feet should be shoulder distance apart.
- Squat down and at the same time raise your arms to chest height.
- Make sure your knees stay over your toes and don't roll inwards.
- Pause and then repeat 10–15 times.

Exercise 25 Sumo squats with balls

Balls are optional; if you don't have them, do the exercise without, or use small water bottles or food cans instead. This is a slight variation on the previous move; it targets your glutes (bottom muscles) and inner thighs.

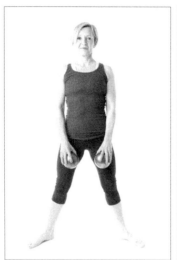 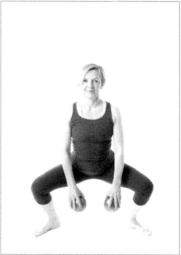

Figure 8.16 (a) Neutral position; (b) Sumo squat holding two balls
– note knees stay wide

- Hold 0.5 kg Pilates balls or small weights in your hands.
- Stand with your knees turned out and feet wide apart.
- Squat down and back, sitting back into your heels – leave your arms hanging down holding the weights.
- Make sure your knees stay wide and don't roll inwards.
- Feel your glutes (buttock muscles) working as you squat.
- Pause and then repeat 10–15 times.

Exercise 26 Bridge with band

You'll need a theraband/resistance band around your lower thighs for this exercise. Choose a light or medium resistance band and place it just above your knees as shown in Figure 8.17.

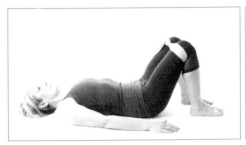 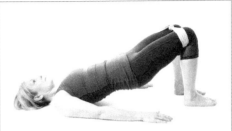

Figure 8.17 (a) Neutral position; (b) Bridge,with band

- Lie on your back, with knees bent, and relax.
- Tighten your deep abdominal muscles – as in Exercise 1, Deep core control (page 105).
- Breathe and relax – but keep the deep engagement in your core.
- Inhale. Then as you exhale, gently tilt your pelvis towards your chest, rolling the imaginary ball to your navel as previously.
- Then allow your bottom to lift and peel your spine of the floor into a low bridge. Don't force your hips too high so it feels uncomfortable. Push through your heels so you get some engagement into your hamstrings and bottom muscles (glutes).
- As you lift up, push your knees outwards into the band. Hold this position for a moment.
- SLOWLY roll back down, one vertebra at a time, and finally untuck your pelvis.
- Relax then repeat the whole process 10–15 times.
- As you get stronger, try to contract your abdominals even tighter throughout the movement.

Exercise 27 Squat with band

You'll need a theraband/resistance band around your lower thighs for this exercise. Choose a light or medium resistance band and place it just above your knees as shown in Figure 8.18.

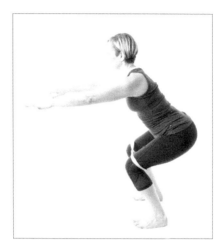

Figure 8.18 Squat with band – note, knees stay over toes

- Stand upright with the band around your thighs just above your knees.
- Your feet should be shoulder distance apart.
- Squat down and at the same time push outwards into the band.
- Make sure your knees stay over your toes and don't roll inwards.
- Pause and then repeat 10–15 times.

Exercise 28 Windmill

This is a nice rotation exercise to help release tightness in your upper/mid spine. You can do it in bed or on the floor.

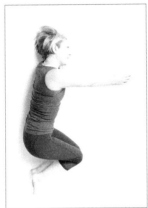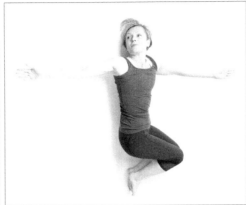

Figure 8.19 (a) Start position; (b) Windmill

- Lie on your left side with your knees tucked up and your arms together out in front of your chest. Have your head supported on a cushion or yoga block.
- Keep your left arm on the floor and your hips facing forward.
- Inhale. Then as you exhale, slowly raise your right arm over and across your body, taking it to the opposite side and towards the floor. Keep your arm slightly bent and aim to get your shoulder to the floor rather than your hand.
- Keep your shoulders down and your hips fixed in position.
- Hold this position, but only go as far as you can manage comfortably. If you've had abdominal surgery, you may not want to stretch too far to begin with, but gradually increase the stretch in time.
- You should feel a stretch across your chest and some stiffness through your mid/upper spine.
- Then slowly return to the start position and repeat 3 times on each side.

Exercise 29 Foam rolling your quads

After bed rest and surgery it's common to be tight in your thigh muscles (quads) and hip flexors. This can give you back and knee pain. Try some gentle self-massage with a foam roller to release your muscles. Start with a soft roller and progress to something harder as you get used to it. Don't underestimate the effectiveness of this exercise.

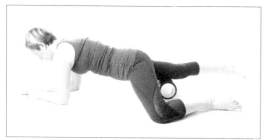 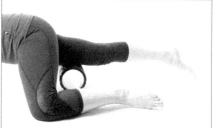

Figure 8.20 (a) and (b) Foam rolling quads

- Lie face down and position the roller under your leg, just above your knee.
- Have your opposite knee bent and out to the side for support.
- Prop yourself up on your elbows and keep your back straight.
- Relax your whole body and breathe.
- Gently and SLOWLY start to work the roller up your thigh – work in short sections and keep going up and down rather than fast rolling.
- Hunt out any tight spots – hover over them and give them some extra work.
- If it's very sore, place your toes on the floor to take some pressure off.
- Spend around 1–2 minutes on each leg.

Exercise 30 Massage ball in glutes

After surgery or bed rest your pelvis and glute (bottom) muscles can feel tight. Gently use a massage ball to release tension. It can make a huge difference to any low back pain. Look for a specific massage ball – a rubber lacrosse ball is ideal; you can find one easily on the internet.

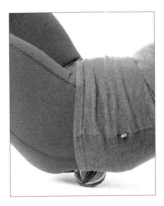

Figure 8.21 Massage ball in glutes

- Prop yourself up on your elbows and place the ball under your glutes as shown in Figure 8.21.
- Gently and slowly move around on the ball and massage any tight spots – keep breathing and move slowly around on the ball.
- Stop and hover over any 'hot spots' and allow them to relax – breathe.
- If this is too much, try pressing up against the wall with the ball wedged between you and the wall.
- Spend 30 seconds to 1 minute on each side and build up.

For those who are more active – returning to sport/formal exercise

This section is aimed at people who want to return to the gym or sporting activities and who are already more active.

As you progress, think about how you move and the surgery you've had. You may want to adapt or modify some moves to take into consideration changes in your body. Even if you've been really fit, don't underestimate the effect of treatment and surgery on your body. Start with these gentle moves before progressing to your usual workouts and sports. Think of this as building your foundations again.

Regulating intra-abdominal pressure (IAP)

As discussed in Chapter 4 (page 44), if you have a stoma or large incision, be cautious of traditional core exercises and learn how to modify or adapt them, especially in the early days. It is generally thought that repeated excessive IAP can increase your risk of hernia around the stoma or an old incision site. Certain movements and exercises can **raise your IAP** and place **undue pressure** on your pelvic floor or abdominal wall. These are to be avoided, at least initially, and include:

- awkward/heavy lifting
- leg press/heavy weighted squats
- breath holding whilst doing an exercise
- isometric bracing positions (where tension is developed without contraction of the muscle), such as planks
- full pull-ups
- cables or activities where the resistance is at the end of a limb
- straight leg sit-ups and crunches with legs raised
- straight leg lifts
- full press-ups
- fit ball roll outs, pikes, hand-roller roll outs etc.

That's not to say never do these exercises again, but be aware of how they feel on your pelvic floor and abdominal wall and adapt or avoid them if they don't feel good. Look out for a feeling of bulging or pressure in your abdomen. If you don't feel in control or you experience any discomfort at all then stop, modify and adapt the exercise.

Ways to modify might include:
- lowering the weight
- improving your breathing technique – don't hold your breath; exhale on the exertion
- doing the same exercise on a weight machine instead of using free weights
- keeping the 'load' closer to the centre of your body
- making exercises more 'isolated' rather than big compound movements (e.g. seated bicep curl rather than a full pull-up)
- do exercises in a supine (on your back) position, rather than prone (facing down).

Using your breath

Using your breath is the first and most important way you can reduce IAP.
- If you want to lift heavy weights in the gym or need to lift heavy things in your work environment, then think about good posture and using your limbs as much as possible to do the work.
- Use your breath to work with you – so you breathe OUT on any lift/exertion. The exhalation has the effect of lowering IAP.
- Try to avoid holding your breath whilst lifting or holding a position.

For example, if you are doing a press-up, you should inhale as you lower your body, then breathe OUT on the part of the movement when you push back UP from the floor. The push UP bit is the 'effort' in this exercise, so breathe out through your mouth as you push up.

In everyday lifting – for example, lifting your dog into the car – bend your knees, get your arms around your dog, then as you lift, think about exhaling and pulling in your abdomen at the same time. Keep the dog close to your body and think about using your arms and legs to do the work.

Classic core exercises – adaptations

In this section I'll show you how to 'modify' some classic core exercises to make them a little safer and to reduce IAP. See also the guidance for specific sports at the end of Chapter 4 (page 48).

Plank

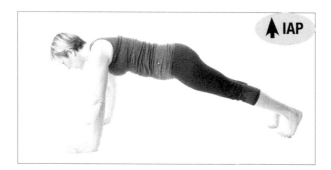

Although they're very popular, I'm not a huge fan of full planks. It's thought that a plank (particularly a full plank on your hands and feet) can place a lot of pressure on the body, increasing IAP and placing downward pressure on the pelvic floor and abdominal wall.

That said, there are many people who like to do them and have no problems. And it can be hard to sit it out if you're in a class setting. So, I've created an 'adaptation' to the plank for people who don't feel comfortable with it, or who have had abdominal surgery, stoma or pelvic surgery or who have a weakened pelvic floor through medication or radiotherapy.

If you've got a hernia or pelvic organ prolapse then you might want to skip the next modified version of a plank also. There are many other ways to safely strengthen your core. But see how it feels. As always, watch out for the feeling of bulging or pressure, in which case stop.

Modified plank

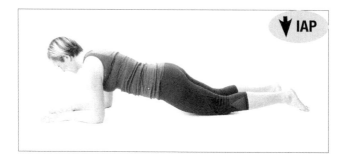

The modified plank is still just as effective, but a little safer and with less pressure. Start lying on your front, elbows under your shoulders, then gently lift your hips a tiny way from the floor until you feel your abdomen working. Do not come any higher. It's just a very gentle hip lift. Keep breathing, lower yourself back down and repeat. Try doing 5–10 repetitions, but only hold each one for a few seconds. Keep breathing.

Crunches

The classic crunch with raised legs and head lifted can place a fair bit of pressure through the abdominal wall and pelvic floor. Notice the abdomen bulging in this figure; modification may be needed.

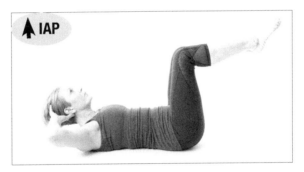

Modified safe curl up

To make this safer, keep your legs straight, engage your deep abdominal muscles, THEN slowly lift your head and shoulders. EXHALE as you lift – the exhalation helps to engage your abdominals and keeps your ribs engaged. Notice how the abdomen in the stoma-safe curl up shown in the Figure below is lying flat without bulging. This subtle change has reduced IAP yet is still effective and works the abdominal muscles in a similar way. Really focus on control and deep muscle engagement and you'll feel it working. Try 10–20 repetitions.

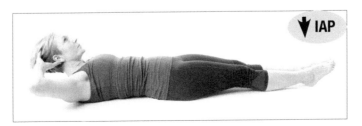

Straight leg lifts or bicycle

Both of these exercises place excessive pressure on the abdominal wall and pelvic floor. You can really see the abdomen bulge in the next two Figures.

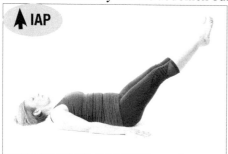 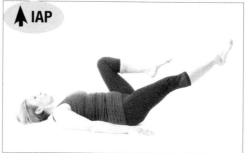

Modified bicycle

To be safer, keep one foot on the floor with your knee bent, the other knee bent, as in the stoma-safe modification in the next figure, and gently curl up either with your hands by your sides or behind your head. This adaptation simply lowers the pressure and means you can do a classic core exercise with a small tweak. Try 10–20 repetitions.

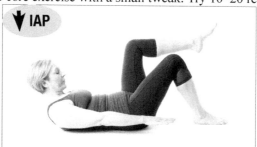

In summary, I am not saying NEVER do any of these exercises, but just start to be aware of the feeling of pressure and how you can adapt a move to make it more appropriate for you. Simple changes can make a huge difference. You can get stronger and build up to some more challenging moves, especially in advanced Pilates or yoga classes, so just feel it out, adapt and modify and get strong before you progress onto anything too challenging.

Putting it all into practice

I appreciate there's a lot to think about and I've given you a lot of exercises to do. Please don't be overwhelmed; there's no need to try and do all of them regularly. Find out which ones work for you, keep them focused and just do what you can manage each day.

Consider your needs and choose exercises specific to you. Do your legs feel weaker than they did? Have you lost a lot of muscle? Do you feel weak through your core/abdominal muscles? Are you worried about your balance and ability to cope with everyday activities? Prioritise exercises to help work on the areas where you feel you need help most.

If you're working with a fitness trainer or physiotherapist, show them this book, ask their advice and get them to help you choose the right moves for you.

Key points

- You don't have to do ALL the exercises from this chapter, just choose the ones that work best for you and mix and match.
- Little and often is best – 3 or 4 times per day. Perhaps choose one exercise to do each hour.
- Some light discomfort/tightness around your surgical site is normal and a feeling of gentle stretching or the muscles working is normal. If you feel strong pain or you ache a lot the following day, then back off or change the exercise you're doing. If an exercise makes pain worse or you're not sure or you have an unusual response, then consult your doctor, nurse or physiotherapist.
- Combine everyday movements with the exercises – so you can multitask – for example, do pelvic floor exercises when sitting in the car or watching TV. You could do squats or sit-stands when waiting for the kettle to boil or marching on the spot when brushing your teeth.
- Try not to think of it as a 'workout' but rather integrate movement into everyday life.
- Chemo and radiotherapy mean a lot of sitting about waiting in hospitals; try to think about the moves you can do when sitting in the waiting room – even if it's just shoulder rolls, core tightening or ankle pumps.

- Just try to move a bit more, even if you don't feel much like it; a bit of gentle movement will help you feel so much better.
- The concept of 'intra-abdominal pressure' is important for anyone who has had abdominal surgery and, in particular, for those who have had a stoma. Watch out for a feeling of bulging or pressure in the abdomen and modify an exercise or activity to reduce the pressure.
- Use a spreadsheet/tracker or notebook to keep a record of the exercises you do and how many you do each day, along with any problems or comments about progression and how good you feel.
- And remember, these mini-exercises form the foundation for future activity, helping to build your confidence and restore movement to your body.

PART IV

DIET AND LIFESTYLE

Chapter 9

Healthy nutrition and hydration

This chapter has been kindly reviewed by Sophie Medlin, Registered Dietitian, who is a specialist in working with people after bowel surgery and with stomas and is director of www.citydietitians.co.uk.

The advice in this chapter is also based on the World Cancer Research Fund nutritional guidelines.[1]

If there's ever a time to really focus on eating well, it's during and after a cancer diagnosis. Nourishing your body with the right nutrients and food can help your body cope with treatment and repair after surgery or chemotherapy, keep your energy levels up and give you the best chance of recovering and living well afterwards.

This is not a time to restrict or remove food groups. This is a time to eat the healthiest, most nourishing food you can. Think about fuelling your body with food that is rich in vitamins and nutrients that your body needs to be healthy.

But, much like exercise, it's one of the hardest times to do it, especially if you're feeling sick, tired or struggling with any digestive issues after surgery. And just like with exercise, there is no 'one rule fits all' solution. Everyone is different when it comes to food choices and responses to surgery and treatment.

So, this chapter is not about eating a specific 'cancer diet' or restricting or eliminating any food groups. It's really just to share some tips on healthy eating and drinking well so that you feel nourished and energised. If you can feel more energised, you'll feel more like being active, so the two things go hand in hand.

Diet and bowel cancer

During cancer and after bowel surgery you will have many questions about what to eat and it can be a confusing time. Search the internet for 'diet and bowel cancer' and you get 12 million results. There is a lot of confusing and conflicting information out there, so trust the advice of your healthcare team and discuss anything you read online with your dietitian and oncology team before making changes.

It's important to keep it simple and focus on a few key points:
1. Focus on nourishing your body for recovery and energy.
2. Reduce your intake of highly processed food.
3. Reduce your intake of sweet foods and added sugar.
4. Eat a diet that includes plenty of fruit, vegetables and grains – in line with World Cancer Research Fund (WCRF) guidelines.
5. Don't restrict any food group – eat a well-balanced diet.
6. Choose foods to stabilise your blood sugar levels.
7. Consume foods high in protein to support recovery and healing.
8. Eat foods to feed your gut health and improve your gut bacteria.
9. Hydrate well – especially if you have a stoma.
10. Know that everyone is different. Eat foods that suit you and that you enjoy.

But what is healthy eating anyway?

There are a lot of myths around diet and nutrition, especially when you have cancer, and it can feel very confusing. This chapter will try to simplify some of the confusing messages and provide some practical advice about what to eat and drink, particularly in relation to exercise and cancer.

This chapter is NOT about specific eating issues, dealing with weight loss or weight gain, problems with food or issues with taste or changes due to chemotherapy or surgery. If you are experiencing these problems, please speak with your nurse or doctor or dietitian.

A 'healthy diet' is generally considered to be one which is low in added sugar and highly processed food. Instead, it is a diet high in fruit, vegetables, protein (meat, fish, nuts, dairy etc) and quality carbohydrates. The WCRF[1] recommends eating a 'plant based' diet for cancer prevention and health during and after cancer treatment. I'll explain what this means a little later.

Eat less highly processed food

Where possible, try to choose food that has not been highly processed, and instead choose food in its most natural state. Cook from scratch where possible and have more homemade meals that include plenty of fruit and vegetables.

Highly processed foods have generally gone through various stages of having 'things' done to them in a factory before they hit the shelves or your plate. Cakes, biscuits, crisps, snacks, breakfast cereals, ready meals, sliced bread, pizza, pastas, shop-bought sandwiches, jars of sauces and things in packets are all examples of highly processed foods. That doesn't mean all of these things are bad or to be completely avoided, it's just about shifting the balance away from eating them all the time and relying on them too heavily.

It's easy to become confused by the arguments about fat, sugar and carbohydrate, when actually all we need to do is take a step back, get the right balance and just eat better quality food and more fruit and vegetables. The *quality and balance* of our diet needs more focus before we start worrying too much about the various components of it.

The 'real food' approach is important for good health in general but also for fuelling your body for the best possible recovery during cancer. That said, when you're not feeling well it can be incredibly hard to cook from scratch or to find foods that you feel like eating. Don't put too much pressure on yourself. It's okay to use pre-packed meals, convenience foods and packet sauces when time is short or if you don't have the energy to cook. Just try not to rely too heavily on overly processed foods; add plenty of fruit and veg and keep things simple.

Why is this important?

Foods that are highly processed are generally lower in fibre, vitamins and other nutrients. They also tend to have a negative effect on your blood sugar levels and energy. They are often higher in salt, additives, sugar and unhealthy fat and can contribute to a wide range of health issues, and prevent you feeling at your best.

Which 'diet' is best for health?

There is no one diet that works for everyone. We're all different and have different needs, likes and dislikes. And that's okay. Try to step away from the confusing dietary advice. Trust your instincts and focus more on your overall eating habits over a longer period of time and your general approach to eating.

That said, one of the most researched diets and the one which comes out consistently best for health is the Mediterranean diet.[2] The Mediterranean diet isn't so much a 'diet' but rather a way of eating, and whilst there are variations from region to region, there are consistent principles.

Unsurprisingly, it's based on eating good quality healthy food that is rich in olive oil, nuts, fish, vegetables, fruit, grains and healthy unsaturated fats. It's generally lower in meat and very low in processed food. Unfortunately, eating a Mediterranean diet doesn't mean lots of pasta and pizza. It has been shown to reduce the risk of heart disease, diabetes, cancer and stroke and fits with the WCRF approach of 'plant based' eating and the 'real food' approach to nutrition.

A plant-based diet means eating mostly foods which come from plants – vegetables, fruit, nuts, seeds, grains and pulses. But it doesn't mean neccesarily being vegetarian or vegan. It's about having the bulk of your food from plants – but also having reasonable amounts of quality meat, fish, dairy.

There are four key reasons for this recommendation.

1. A plant-based diet can help you stay a healthy weight – being a healthy weight is thought to reduce your risk of many chronic conditions, including cancer.
2. Vegetables and fruit provide vitamins, minerals and something called 'phytochemicals' which help protect cells in the body from damage that can lead to cancer. Different types of fruit and veg provide different types of phytochemicals, so it's important to eat a wide variety every day.
3. A diet high in fibre (whole grains, fruit and veg) has been shown to reduce the risk of bowel cancer and can get your bowel healthy again after surgery.
4. Gut health and the microbiome (see page 162) are one of the most interesting and emerging areas of health research – linked with a reduction in cancer risk, diabetes, heart disease and other chronic health conditions, as well as appetite and obesity. A diet high in fibre, vegetables and wholegrains will help to feed the right kinds of bacteria in your bowel and, in my view, this is one of the most compelling reasons to eat plant-based foods.

What about five-a-day?

You've heard it hundreds of times but eating at least five portions of fruit and vegetables each day really is one of the simplest, yet most important, steps you can take to improve your health – reducing your risk of heart disease, cancer, diabetes and many other chronic conditions.

But most of us still don't eat enough fruit and vegetables. The average person in the UK is thought to eat approximately 3–4 portions per day, so there's plenty of work to do. In Australia, the recommended amount is five vegetables and two fruit portions per day (a total of seven portions per day), and it's likely that other countries will soon follow the same recommendation.

It doesn't have to be difficult, but it might require a bit of planning on your part and a bit of effort if it's not something you already do. There are easy ways to sneak fruit and veg into your diet, including smoothies and adding fruit to breakfast cereal etc. And when meal planning, choose your vegetables first, then plan the rest of your meal around them.

A 'portion' of fruit or vegetables is considered to be about 80 g – for example, a medium banana, large apple, large orange, five florets of broccoli, a small bag of spinach or a bowl of mixed salad. Have something at every meal and spread out your five portions throughout the day. Berries on your breakfast, carrot sticks mid-morning, salad at lunch, banana mid-afternoon and steamed vegetables at dinner, for example.

To get the widest range of phytochemicals and nutrients, think about eating a rainbow of colours each and every day. Red berries, yellow bananas or sweetcorn, orange fruit, red melon, green watercress and spinach, blueberries – you get the picture. As much variety as possible is the goal. Some dietitians recommend aiming for 30 different types of fruits, vegetables, seeds, nuts, grains and plants over the course of a week.

After bowel surgery or stoma

It's super-important to increase your fruit and vegetable intake, but it can be hard if you've just had bowel surgery or you have digestive problems. If you've been advised to eat a soft/low-residue diet (generally this is based on low-fibre, higher-energy foods that are easy to digest), think about how to prepare or cook fruit and vegetables differently. You'll still get the same nutrients and benefits, but with less fibre. (But always speak with you nurse or dietitian about your own personal nutrition needs.)

Here are some examples.

- Rather than a raw apple, cook apples into a purée and eat with custard or yoghurt.
- Instead of eating a banana raw, can you turn it into a banana and peanut butter milkshake in the blender.

• Raw veg and salad can be hard to digest: could you sauté your spinach and have tender cooked vegetables instead?

As with exercise, instead of saying 'I can't', find alternative ways to say 'I can', and cook with a bit of creative thinking and food preparation.

Sugar

Most people consume far too much sugary food and it's fuelling ill-health on many levels. No-one would argue that consuming too much 'added sugar' is a good thing. However, we are in danger of going too far in the opposite direction and making sugar into the enemy. This makes us fearful of eating anything sweet and that's equally damaging. No-one should be worrying about eating a piece of fruit.

Sugar is only part of the picture and there are many foods that are higher in naturally occurring sugars that do provide nutrients and vitamins which are good for us. Fruit is a great example; although high in naturally occurring sugars, it's also healthy and packed full of phytonutrients, and we should be eating plenty of it.

During and after cancer treatment, it becomes even more important to eat well with a wide range of nourishing foods. Fuel your body with as much nourishment as possible, rather than be too restrictive. Make every calorie count and think about what that food is providing for your body.

Keep things in balance and avoid demonising all sugars in the same way. No-one should feel guilty about having a cake from time to time, or a chocolate bar or pudding. Not if it's part of an otherwise healthy and balanced diet. This comes back to the basic concept of cutting down on the processed stuff. If you do that, you'll automatically cut down on refined/added sugar.

Biscuits, sweets, cakes, breakfast cereals, sugary drinks and snacks are all high in processed refined sugar, but lacking in fibre and nutrition, and basically provide very little of the 'nourishment' we all desperately need. They can also create havoc with your blood sugar levels and energy, making it difficult to be active, sleep well, concentrate and function in life. It makes sense to try to reduce your intake of refined sugar, but not cut it out entirely, and choose foods where sugar occurs naturally, such as in fruit or vegetables.

Stabilise your blood sugar levels

One of the key reasons to reduce your reliance on sugar is to help stabilise your blood sugar levels. This is especially important if you're feeling unwell, tired and fatigued during treatment or when recovering from cancer. Stable blood sugar levels will also help you to be more active and feel more energised. Choosing foods that provide slow-release energy will help stabilise your blood sugar levels more effectively, rather than the 'crash and burn' feeling you'll get after sugar or too much carbohydrate.

Symptoms of this are the 'afternoon slump', headaches, low levels of concentration, feeling hungry all the time, feeling a crash in energy not long after eating a meal and feeling light headed if you haven't eaten for a while. If that sounds familiar, then try swapping high-sugar foods for slower release/quality carbohydrates (such as wholemeal grains, sweet potato, high-fibre foods etc.) and more protein and fat.

Cancer treatments may affect your blood sugar levels too, and you may find you have big swings and slumps in energy, so talk with your nurse or doctor about this and pay even more attention to your diet to try to include appetite-stabilising foods, less sugar and regular meals.

Here are some top tips to stabilise your blood sugar levels.

- Start by cutting out sugar in your tea and coffee – reduce by half a teaspoon at a time. And don't swap sugar for artificial sweetener, as it won't 'reset' your taste for sugar. You need to re-educate your palate to enjoy less-sweet foods and drinks.
- Drinks like fizzy drinks, bottled smoothies, sports drinks, pop, soda and fruit juices might give you an instant energy kick but are loaded with sugar. Instead have plain water or diluted fruit juice.
- Include a source of protein in every meal – eggs, natural yoghurt, nuts, meat, fish, chicken, pulses and beans. Protein slows down the release of energy, giving you more stable blood sugar levels, and you'll feel fuller for longer. Instead of a processed breakfast cereal (such as cornflakes) to start the day – which will have you wanting more sugar by mid-morning – have something like scrambled eggs and rye bread instead. See how much more energy you've got as a result.
- One of the best pieces of advice given to me by my surgeon after my bowel surgery, was to use a protein powder supplement 2–3 times per day. I could digest it easily and it helped me recover, rebuild my muscle and repair tissue after the surgery. I use whey isolate natural protein powder even now in a

breakfast smoothie (see page 199 for details of brand).

- Don't be scared of fat. The tables have turned after decades of misleading advice, and we're now realising the importance of including healthy fat in our diet – it has an appetite-stabilising effect but also binds to essential vitamins and other nutrients. This also fits with the Mediterranean approach to eating. Including foods in their most natural state, such as avocado, nuts, oils and seeds, which are really good for you, and choosing full-fat dairy foods such as Greek yoghurt, full-fat milk and cheese. These are all far better choices than low-fat, processed alternatives, which are often higher in sugar. Nourishing, simple, natural food is what it's all about.

- Eating regularly and planning ahead will help manage your blood sugar levels, especially during treatment. If you're planning to exercise or do something more active, have a snack or small meal about 1–2 hours beforehand – include some protein, carbohydrate (wholegrains, fruit or vegetables) and a small amount of fat. Things like peanut butter on a slice of rye bread, or a banana smoothie made with milk, are good pre-exercise snacks.

- Carry snacks and a drink with you if you're out and about – things such as nuts, fruit, protein balls etc. Planning ahead will stop you from picking up cakes, biscuits, sweets and sugary drinks.

- Aim to have at least one proper meal each day. Sometimes it's easier to graze and snack all day, but one larger meal will make you feel more satisfied and energised. Fill in the rest of the day with other snacks and small meals.

- Dairy foods – milk, yoghurt and cheese – are important. They provide calcium which is needed for bone strength. Chemotherapy and hormone drugs can affect your bone strength, so it's important to do all you can for your bone health. Have full-fat versions and enjoy a smaller amount. It's far better to have all-natural full-fat Greek yoghurt instead of a fat-free sweetened yoghurt full of sugar and artificial additives.

Gut microbiome

One of the most interesting areas of research in health at the moment is in 'gut health'. Scientists have discovered that the gut – particularly the large intestine – contains bacteria (colonic bacteria) which are incredibly important for both our mental and physical health. The bacteria are thought to be so important that it's almost like having a second brain.

It's thought that the gut contains somewhere between 300 and 400 trillion microorganisms and this diverse and well-populated gut microbiome helps us prevent and fight a whole range of diseases, including cancer. The bacteria keep our immune system strong and help with mood problems, joint pain, inflammation, obesity and appetite, and skin complaints.

Although it's early days, some new research[3] is also beginning to look at the link between cancer and the gut microbiome. Some early studies have shown that people with healthy gut bacteria respond better to immunotherapy, and other studies have shown some people who develop colon cancer have less diverse bacteria – in other words, having a healthy gut microbiome could potentially be protective against colon cancer.

Developing this research further could mean manipulating the gut microbiome to help prevent and treat cancer, or to help immunotherapy drugs work better, as having a healthy gut microbiome seems to create an anti-inflammatory response in the body. It's too early to say where this research will lead, but it shows promise for both cancer prevention and treatment. If you want to read more about it have a look at the website www.cancerresearchuk.org and search for 'gut microbiome'.

Our gut microbiome needs to take priority for our current and future health. Forget about restrictive low-carbohydrate or high-fat diets. A restricted low-carb diet/high-fat or keto diet (a diet low in carbohydrate and high in fat) could mean you can't get enough fibre from wholegrains and plants to feed your gut bacteria. To improve gut health we are back to the concept of a balanced plant-based diet, with plenty of fruit and veg, little processed food/sugar and lots of fibre. Not exactly rocket science. But now you know exactly WHY it's important.

So how do you improve your gut microbiome?

But our guts aren't as healthy or happy as they should be. Our modern lifestyles, poor diet choices, highly processed foods, high-sugar intake, antibiotic use and low-fibre diets all contribute to a gut microbiome that isn't as diverse and healthy as it could be, and this is affecting our health in a really significant way. After bowel cancer and surgery, we need to give our guts as much help as we can and restore the healthy bacteria.

We can do a lot to improve our gut health. If there's ever a reason to eat vegetables, this is it. Eating a wide range of plant foods is the foundation of having a healthy gut. Especially vegetables such as broccoli and cauliflower and foods that have plenty of fibre – wholegrains, nuts, pulses and beans. These foods act like a 'fertiliser' and get the gut bacteria growing in the first place.

Eating processed foods high in refined sugar, does the opposite and reduces our gut microbiome diversity. Another great reason to ditch the junk food and sugar. For optimum gut health you need to attack it from all angles – reduce sugar and processed foods, increase fibre, vegetables and whole grains, and try using fermented foods such as live yoghurt.

It's a new and exciting area of nutrition, so do some more reading around it and find out how you might benefit.

Some diet challenges

After bowel surgery and stoma surgery

If you've had surgery to remove a section of your bowel or all of your colon, and/or a stoma, eating a diet high in fibre and plants can be a bit more difficult, especially if you have a specific type of stoma called an ileostomy (see Chapter 4).

A diet high in fibre, fruit and veg is often the opposite of what people are advised to eat after bowel/stoma surgery. However, the gut does adapt and in time you should be able to introduce a wider range of foods and eat a normal healthy diet, potentially with a few adaptations. It's important not to feel 'fear' about any food or to label foods as good/bad. Experiment and find what works for you.

People who don't have their large intestine anymore and have a stoma still need to give focus to eating fibre – as foods high in fibre contain other important nutrients – but you need to take a slightly different approach. The recommended daily amount of fibre is 30 g for the normal population, but if you have an ileostomy it may be difficult (and unnecessary) to try to achieve that amount.

Although nothing should be restricted or avoided, you may need to take more care with foods which are harder to digest. Only through trial and error (hopefully not too much error) will you know what suits you.

The problem is that everyone is different and can tolerate different foods. It's generally not a specific food that causes an issue in someone with a stoma, but the amount of it. A couple of nuts won't cause a problem, but a whole bag might. And similarly, a small salad with lunch might be fine, but a huge salad with lots of raw vegetables at lunch AND dinner on the same day might be too much, leaving you feeling uncomfortable or even with a blockage. All you can do is try small amounts of new foods at a time, monitor how they go through and see how you feel.

However, making an effort to eat a wide range of healthy foods and a plant-based diet is still super-important even if you have a stoma. Gut health is the priority here, along with making sure you get enough nutrients from a healthy well-balanced diet. You just have to figure out some adaptations and cook/prepare foods in a different way. Speak to your stoma nurse for more advice or contact a specialist dietitian who works closely with stoma patients.

If you have an ileostomy and have had your colon removed no-one knows for sure how the gut microbiome is impacted and what effect this has on wider health. Hopefully this will be an area of research in the near future.

Other eating problems and disorders

When you're going through treatment or after bowel surgery, your appetite can change, and you can have symptoms which make it difficult to eat and drink, so eating can become challenging in general. You might also experience weight gain or weight loss and your relationship with food can change significantly. That's beyond the scope of this chapter, but there are some excellent resources for 'eating problems' during cancer online at WCRF,[4] and the National Cancer Institute.[5]

Please contact a specialist oncology dietitian if you have specific issues or need advice.

Our relationship with food is complex at the best of times and a bowel cancer diagnosis and treatment can disrupt it to the point of disordered eating. Whilst there isn't much research connecting cancer and stoma surgery to eating disorders, they are becoming more common across all age groups and are often triggered by changes in body shape, appetite, surgery and after illness. If you feel that your relationship with food is changing, you're becoming too restrictive and you need support, then please ask for a referral to a therapist or counsellor with skills in treating disordered eating. Also contact BEAT – the charity for eating disorders (see page 199).

Hydration

Most of the population in the UK are walking around in a chronic mildly dehydrated state most of the time. It's thought that around 80% of us don't drink enough for good health on a day-to-day basis. Headaches, grogginess, fatigue, nausea, low energy, feeling thirsty and an inability to concentrate are all symptoms of not drinking enough water. Just being dehydrated by 1–2% of your body weight can reduce your ability to concentrate and you can feel quite groggy and fatigued.

During a normal day the typical body loses around 2–2.5 litres of fluid – through sweating, breathing and waste leaving the body. If the weather is hot or you exercise and sweat more, you'll lose more fluid. During exercise it's possible to lose between 0.5 and 2 litres of fluid. Air conditioning and flying add to fluid losses even more. You can see how easy it is for these to stack up.

If you're sick from chemotherapy, have diarrhoea or a fever or are not feeling well – and therefore not drinking enough and losing more fluid – you can quickly end up severely dehydrated. More serious effects of dehydration include low blood pressure, fainting, confusion and rapid heartrate. Contact your GP or nurse if you experience these symptoms.

If you have had your large intestine (colon) removed and you have an ileostomy, your body will need even more salts and fluids. People with an ileostomy can lose an additional 1000–1500 ml of fluid per day, and this needs to be replaced with an electrolyte drink.

Avoid drinking lots of plain water as this can flush the electrolytes from your body even more. You need a drink which includes the correct balance of salts, glucose and fluid and choose to have this on a daily basis, to prevent dehydration (see page 199 for recommendations).

Drink electrolyte drinks every day (start with 200–400 ml, although you may need as much as 1 litre), along with a mixed fluid intake from tea, coffee, soft drinks, water and juices etc. Speak to your GP, stoma nurse or a dietitian if you need more advice.

However, for the majority of people, a little extra effort increasing fluid intake can have a transformational effect on how they feel.

Case study

Stuart came into my exercise group and we started with some easy walking on the treadmill. He had had chemo treatment the previous week and had been vomiting, but was feeling much better now. However, within just a few minutes he said he felt dizzy and seconds later he rolled onto the floor feeling unwell. His blood pressure was low and it took numerous attempts over the next hour to get him back up to sitting, and then finally standing up. After a check-over from the

---

doctor, he was absolutely fine and he didn't need any treatment, but he needed some snacks and a drink to get him back up.

What had happened? That morning Stuart had been feeling tired, so he'd stayed in a warm bed until 12 noon, without drinking or eating, then came straight to exercise. On top of being sick the previous week, the result was that he was chronically dehydrated and under-fuelled for exercise. As soon as he started to exercise his blood pressure dropped, causing him to feel unwell.

This experience taught Stuart a lot. He realised that if he wanted to continue coming to exercise group he would need a new strategy. The following week he got up earlier, had plenty to drink and ate some breakfast about 2 hours before his gym session. In the 24 hours beforehand he made an effort to drink more too. Unsurprisingly he felt much better, more energised and able to exercise.

What surprised Stuart most was that feeling quite unwell was simply due to dehydration and not eating enough. A few tweaks to his diet and hydration strategy and he felt much better.

The risk of dehydration is higher for people with cancer, but there's plenty you can do to help yourself. Here is a list of things to look out for and what to do if you are getting dehydrated.

- Be aware of any symptoms of mild dehydration – dry lips, tongue, feeling thirsty, fatigue, grogginess, dark urine, dizziness etc – and stay one step ahead.
- Monitor your urine colour – it should be the colour of pale straw. Be really honest when you inspect it. If it's any darker (darker yellow) or strong smelling, then it's a sure sign you're dehydrated, and you need to drink more.
- If your urine colour is very pale and almost clear, you could be drinking too much – or having inconsistent volumes throughout the day. Get the balance right. Aim for pale straw-coloured urine rather than colourless.
- Make it a habit to drink more during the day – carry a bottle with you everywhere, aim to drink small amounts regularly throughout the day.
- Drink before you're thirsty. By the time you feel thirsty, the chances are you'll already be dehydrated. Get into the habit of drinking regularly before

you feel you really need it.

- Aim to have a mixed fluid intake. Tea, coffee, water, milk, juice and squash all count towards your fluid intake, but try to reduce sugary drinks as much as possible.
- Add flavour to water with pieces of fruit such as slices of lemon or orange.
- Remember that everyone is different – some people will need 2 litres of fluid per day (or more), some will need less. It depends on your own personal fluid losses and needs.
- So instead of aiming for '8 glasses' or 2 litres of fluid, which is often the standard advice, use your urine colour and symptoms to monitor your own hydration status and drink more, or less.
- What you drink in the 12–24 hours prior to an exercise session will have far more impact on what you drink DURING it. Start exercise well hydrated by drinking plenty in advance.
- If it's hot or you're exercising for more than 1 hour, then you will need additional fluid during exercise. Use a sports bottle and drink little and often.
- And finally… consider using electrolyte drinks rather than plain water both during exercise and if you have an ileostomy. It can be like a turbo boost. The combination of sodium and glucose helps your body absorb fluid better and replaces lost salts.
- Avoid sugary sports drinks (such as Lucozade or similar) and make your own by adding a pinch of salt to dilute squash, or if you have a lot of fluid losses, then use an oral rehydration solution such as Dioralyte. Speak to your doctor or nurse about this.

Key points

- The concept of nourishing your body with good food is essential when you have cancer. Avoid restrictive diets and removing food groups, in particular carbohydrates. When you're at your most vulnerable is the time you need to fuel your body with quality food and lots of fruit and vegetables. This will give your body the best chance of healing and recovery.
- Reduce your intake of highly processed food. Try to avoid cakes, crisps, pre-packed meals, sandwiches, biscuits, breakfast cereals and white carbs. If you can, aim for more home-cooked nourishing meals and plenty of fruit and vegetables.
- Reduce your intake of sweet foods and added sugar. This will help to stabilise your blood sugar levels. Elevated blood sugar levels are related to chronic inflammation in the body and many chronic health conditions, such as cancer, heart disease and stroke. Equally, there's no need to go 'sugar free' or to turn sugar into the 'devil'; just keep things in balance and avoid 'added' sugar, sweet drinks and too many processed sweet foods.
- Although obvious, it's vital to eat a diet that includes plenty of fruit, vegetables and grains – in line with WCRF guidelines. Yet many of us still struggle to get our '5 a day'. Think of ways to 'sneak' fruit and veg into your diet, especially if you're struggling with digestive issues. Homemade smoothies are great and you can add avocados, spinach, berries and nuts to create a really balanced 'liquid meal'.
- Although it's popular to eat a low-carb diet, cutting out carbohydrates can have a negative effect on your gut health and blood sugar levels. Instead of cutting them out altogether, choose quality wholemeal grains and high fibre sources of carbohydrates, rather than white pasta, rice and white bread.
- Protein is super-important during treatment and beyond to help your body heal and recovery. Include a source of protein (meat, fish, eggs, nuts etc) at each meal. If you find that hard due to digestive issues, add natural protein powder to smoothies or to porridge, yoghurt or soup.
- 'Gut health' are the buzzwords of the moment and for good reason.

169

A healthy gut microbiome is linked to lower body weight, better mental wellbeing, lower risk of cancer, heart disease and other chronic conditions, and the research is very exciting. The importance of eating a diet to improve our gut microbiome is super-important, choosing plenty of fruit and veg, fibre and a wide range of foods, including nuts and seeds. It's so much more than just taking a probiotic. I urge you to read more about it and look at how you can improve your own gut microbiome.

- Hydration goes hand in hand with feeling well enough to exercise. Most people are chronically dehydrated and not drinking enough for good health. This leads to fatigue and a feeling of grogginess, headaches and tiredness. Really focus on increasing your fluid intake and see how much better you feel, and if you have a stoma or regularly have diarrhoea, include an oral rehydration solution in your daily fluid intake.

- Everyone is different. There is no one rule that fits all, even when you have cancer, and especially after bowel surgery. Find foods that you enjoy, that you feel nourish you and work with your digestive system. It can be harder to eat a healthy diet during and after bowel cancer, but not impossible; it just takes a little extra effort. But the effort will pay off as you'll enjoy increased energy, more stable blood sugar levels and a healthier digestive system for the future.

Chapter 10

Overcoming barriers and getting motivated

The advice and information in this book might well be useful, informative and motivational, but 'knowing' and 'doing' are two completely different things.

I'm thrilled you've got this far, but how do you get from 'I know I should do some exercise' to doing it and putting it into practice. That's often much harder. Changing behaviour is tough at the best of times, but when you're thrown the 'cancer curve ball' it can seem impossible.

We all have barriers – things that stop us from doing something. They might be real or perceived and are often connected with our emotions, fears and lack of knowledge or support. They can also be based on what we've heard from someone else, particularly a healthcare professional or another patient. Barriers are different for all of us and how we deal with a challenge is psychological and tied into previous experiences and something called 'self-efficacy' – a term psychologists use to describe how confident we are about our ability to do something.

Common barriers to exercise for most people are things like 'I don't have time' or 'I'm too tired'. Even when you feel well and healthy it's not difficult to find excuses not to be active, or to put it off until tomorrow. When you have cancer there are many more barriers and they can seem insurmountable at times. Pain, fear about harming yourself, cancer-related fatigue, anxiety, depression, not knowing what to do, being told to rest. The list goes on.

When it comes to exercise, many of us have barriers and obstacles to overcome. It's natural to find excuses when something is difficult, or we find it hard, or we don't have experience or knowledge of how to handle it. But ironically, during and after cancer is the time when you actually need it the most. It's the time when you need to dig deep to find ways to overcome these challenges. Invest time, effort and energy into finding solutions to the obstacles and ways around the barriers. It might not be easy, but the benefits will be enormous.

You'll know from reading the earlier chapters in this book that exercise is safe both during and after treatment. You should also have some idea of a timeline after surgery and ways to monitor your exercise intensity and recovery. All of these things are important to know but now it's time to think more deeply and identify where your barriers are and how you put 'knowledge' into action.

> **Case study**
>
> Emma is a young woman in her 20s who came along to a workshop I gave to a cancer charity. We were talking about barriers to exercise and Emma said that she used to love going to Zumba. But now she had had chemo, had lost her hair and wore a wig, she felt self-conscious and got hot when she exercised. This meant that she wasn't going to her fitness dance class anymore and was missing out on something she loved.
>
> Her mum did some research and found a 'disco' fitness class at her local centre which used glow sticks and, most importantly, was in the dark! Emma nervously went along and took off her wig, danced with her glow sticks at the back where no-one could see her (because it was dark) and loved every second.
>
> This is a brilliant example of 'growth mindset'... instead of saying 'I can't', Emma chose to say, 'Okay so how can I do this differently?' Rather than seeing a barrier, Emma (along with the help from her mum) saw an alternative and a way around the problem.

What are YOUR barriers?

Now it's time to work through your barriers and obstacles and look at ways you can get around them. Some common ones are listed in the table opposite.

Barrier/problem/ obstacle	Solution
Haven't got time. Am so busy with hospital appointments and trying to juggle work and family as well	Could I walk to the hospital? Or at least part of the way? Get my partner to drop me off 15 mins walk away while they find a parking spot?
I'm so tired and really don't feel like it	I have to remind myself that the best way to relieve cancer-related fatigue is with exercise. I know I feel better if I make myself do something, even it's just for 10 minutes. I'll ask my friend to take me for a walk and we'll put it in the diary, even if I don't feel like it. Is something else making me tired? Am I dehydrated? Or not eating enough? What can I do about it?
I really don't enjoy the gym and exercise	Gardening, walking, DIY and vigorous housework are great ways to exercise. I don't have to go to the gym to be active. How can I turn my gardening into something a bit more active? Can I do some step-ups and dig a bit more vigorously?
My family are all telling me to rest	I will ask them to support me to be active instead, show them this book and ask them to encourage me to walk or go for a swim or bike ride and to come with me.
I have good intentions to go for a walk or jog, but it never seems to happen	I could ask a friend to come with me. Putting it in the diary will commit us both. Can I join a walking group or running group? They have set session times, which means I'm more likely to go. Can I offer to walk next door's dog? That way I'm committed and will have to do it.
I've got lymphoedema/ neuropathy/a stoma/ just had surgery	There's always something you can do. If you've just had surgery, do your rehab exercises which will rebuild your confidence. If you find walking difficult because of balance problems, then try cycling or swimming instead. You may have a limitation but what CAN you do?
I'm in pain	What's causing the pain? Does exercise make it worse or better? What can I do to make it better? What exercise can I do despite it? Long-term chronic pain is also often connected with our emotions and fatigue, and can become a vicious circle.

You may recognise some of the reasons for not exercising listed in the table on page 173.

Complete a table for yourself. Think about some of the things that stop you from being active – things that make it difficult for you. Write down 3–4 things that you feel get in the way of your being active right now in the table below. They might be related to your cancer, or they might not. You might have more than 3–4 things. That's okay too, just write it all down; either here or in a separate notebook.

Barrier/problem/obstacle	Solution

Then start to break down those barriers. This may require a bit of deep thought and unpicking. For each thing you've written down in the left-hand column, go through the following list and write a response in the right-hand column as to how you could overcome the corresponding barrier.

- Do you need any more information, treatment or advice? (from a doctor, physio or nurse) about a cancer-specific issue or to treat a musculoskeletal problem?
- Can you do exercise in a different way? If an exercise bike is uncomfortable, can you use a stepper machine or try a recumbent bike? Or try a different saddle?
- Can you *think* about it in a different way? Take a different approach? Instead of one long walk, can you do two short walks in a day instead?
- What research/communications do you need to do? Find out times of classes or sessions? Message a friend? Book a session with a trainer? Join a gym or pay a membership?
- Is there anything you need to purchase? Clothing? New trainers? A fitness

tracker? A piece of exercise equipment? An app for your phone?

- Is there anything practical you need to do? Perhaps move furniture around so you have an exercise space?
- What do you need to do to make it happen? Break it down, step by step.
- Do you have contingency plans? Can you adjust the time, intensity and volume if you're feeling great? If the weather is bad, do you have waterproofs or an alternative? Keep your options open.

It's important that you do this exercise yourself. Coming up with your own solutions is much more empowering and motivating than someone else doing it for you. Give this exercise some time and thought… you might need to return to it a couple of times.

And then for each of the barriers, focus on the benefits. What will you GAIN from overcoming this barrier? What is the benefit for you?

Here's the table again, with an example filled in to get you started.

Barrier/problem/ obstacle	Solutions	Benefit
Feeling too tired to exercise	Ask my daughter to take me for a 10-minute walk to the end of the road and back Use the 'Active 10' App on my phone to remind me to walk	Walking will energise me and help me feel LESS tired later on. Having the company of my daughter will be nice too and will motivate me if I can't face it I'll feel a sense of achievement and will set a goal of doing 2 x 10 minutes each day. I'll feel more energised and I'll sleep better

Who's your support crew?

Most of us do better if we exercise with someone else or in a group. Just arranging to do an activity with someone else means we're more likely to turn up.

By making a commitment, there's accountability to another person. Booking a class or session, or agreeing to meet a friend, means you'll have a set appointment to attend, upping the chances of your making it happen. You're less likely to make an excuse if you have to explain it to someone else. And having the support of someone else is hugely important – someone who can encourage you when you otherwise might find it tough to get going. You need friends and family to be the voice of 'Come on, you can do this'… rather than 'Oh dear, you need to rest'.

Research has also shown that exercising with a friend or in a group reduces feelings of fatigue and pain (compared with exercising on your own) and you're more likely to do it for longer. In addition, the mood-boosting, stress-reducing effects of exercise are enhanced when you exercise with a friend or partner.

So, who can help you? Who's your support crew? It might be a friend, a nurse, or support group, an exercise group or class, family or even an animal. Anyone in your life who provides support, encouragement and an opportunity for you to be active. They might not be in your life yet, so there's an opportunity to do some research, find groups, people and sessions that can help you.

Make a list – who are my support crew?

1.

2.

3.

4.

5.

And if you don't have anyone in your support crew, where can you find them? It doesn't have to be a cancer-specific group or a health professional. Could you join a supportive walking group? How about a friend from a cancer support group? Could you go for a walk instead of sitting having a coffee? Could you ask your neighbours if you could walk their dog? Ask your close family to support you to be active, rather than them encouraging you to rest. You may need to be clear about what you need from them.

Next, make a list of ways in which each person/support crew can help. Can you schedule to do things together? Ask for their help and share your ideas. Together you can help each other. This might be things like meeting you at the gym, going for a walk instead of a coffee, joining you to do a Pilates class or booking a personal trainer or class.

How can my support crew help me?

1.

2.

3.

4.

5.

Re-think your recovery mindset

We generally expect recovery to be a linear process. We think we have our treatment or surgery and then when it's over, each day gets better than the last. We have surgery/treatment. We recover and then finally we 'get back to normal'. Unfortunately, it doesn't work like that. Living with cancer is far from linear.

There are good days and there are bad days and, with cancer especially, every day is different. Once you can adapt to that new way of thinking and learn to go with the flow, it becomes easier to cope. Learning to be flexible and accepting are essential new tools in your emotional armoury.

Living with cancer isn't easy and it can feel like a roller coaster at times. But having one bad day doesn't mean you're going backwards; it just means you're having a bad day. Know that tomorrow will probably be better. When you look at the overall picture, you'll see it's a journey of ups and downs, hopefully going in the right direction (see Figure 10.1). Try not to focus on a final 'destination', or on where you've been. Just focus on today and the 'now'. Mindfulness training can help with this, or even some counselling or therapy.

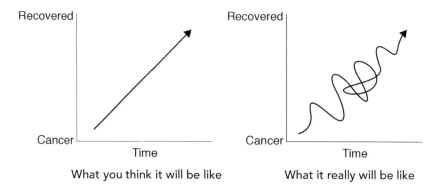

Figure 10.1 The cancer recovery pathway is never straightforward
(based on an idea by physiotherapist Adam Meakins)

Ideas for activities

Movement, physical activity and exercise

Go back to something I mentioned in Chapter 1 about the differences between 'exercise', 'physical activity' and 'movement' (see Figure 10.2).

- 'Exercise' is defined as being purposeful and something that you might do with the aim of getting fit or improving your health. There is a clear goal and purposeful intention. Some examples might be going for a run or going to the gym.
- 'Physical activity' is defined as something that involves bodily movement *as a consequence rather than as a goal*. So, some good examples of this might be walking to work or doing some gardening or housework.
- 'Movement' is just that. Literally any kind of bodily movement involving the musculoskeletal system. This might simply be taking regular breaks from sitting at your computer or TV, or walking around your house, climbing stairs or just not being 'sedentary'.

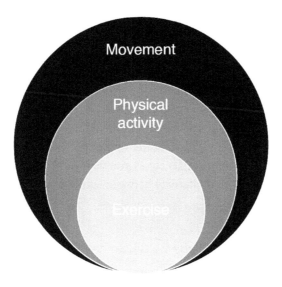

Figure 10.2 The relationship between exercise, physical activity and movement

So how do you translate this into real life?

In an ideal world, we need to focus on all three areas for optimum health benefits. Although any sort of movement – no matter how small – is brilliant.

Simply, just try to sit less. Then start to include more structured physical activity and exercise into your life. There are literally hundreds of options. Here are some ideas.

Movement snacks

Movement snacks are exactly how they sound. Tiny burst of movement throughout your day. These are not formal exercise sessions, but are ways of being more active, breaking up long periods of sitting.

- Set an alarm on your phone or watch to remind you to move every 60 minutes – get up, stretch, do 10 'sit stands' (page 138) or 20 'calf raises' (page 135) and walk up and down your stairs.
- Drink more fluid, which will make you walk to the loo more often.
- When travelling in the car or on a train/plane, take regular breaks – get up and move around. Stretch, move and walk whenever you get the chance.
- Design your own 'movement snack' programme using the exercises in Chapters 7 and 8 – tick them off when you do them. Try to do something every hour.

- Don't watch TV or films passively – sitting in the same position for an hour or more. Use the opportunity to stretch, sit on the floor, move positions and do some core exercises.
- Be a 'chair rebel' – when someone offers you a seat in a waiting room or meeting, do the opposite – politely decline and stand instead.
- Multi-task activities such as waiting for a kettle to boil, putting fuel in the car or brushing your teeth – they all offer opportunities for stretches, calf raises, shoulder rotations, mini squats etc as you wait.
- Get a standing desk and alternate between sitting and standing during the day when you're working.

Monitor your daily physical activity

Invest in an activity tracker to wear on your wrist (they're a bit like a watch – see page 198 for details) that counts your daily steps and distance. You can get a model which measures heartrate too. Using a step tracker device has been shown to be effective in increasing physical activity levels in people after a cancer diagnosis and it can be motivational, especially if you have a model which 'nudges' you to move after periods of sitting.

There are two ways to use an activity tracker:
- Daily step count – forget the 10,000-step target, which is often unrealistic for many. Instead, just take a note of your daily step count and try to increase it by small amounts each day. Over time you can increase your walking frequency, distance and intensity.
- Heartrate – calculate your heartrate target (using the methods outlined in Chapter 6) and use the monitor to make sure you get your exercise intensity right. You can do this if you're walking or jogging.

Cancer exercise class/exercise referral group

Ask your oncologist or nurse if there is a cancer-specific exercise group at your hospital, hospice or local gym or in the community. They are few and far between, but where they do exist, they offer a supportive, safe, supervised and encouraging environment – usually a circuit-style class or sometimes walking groups. You might also find you can access a 'GP or exercise referral class' (which are for people with medical conditions) – these are usually at your local leisure centre and are heavily subsidised, so the cost is low. You can either ask your GP to refer you or, more frequently, you can self-refer to a group.

Community/gym exercise group or class

There are hundreds of different types of classes/groups in the local community or at local gyms. so you're bound to find something to suit. From Tai Chi to tennis, Zumba to running, Pilates to water aerobics, walking to cycling – find a group, club or class that is welcoming to all, isn't competitive and provides a friendly supportive environment.

Of course, if you're already fit, then you can probably continue with classes, sessions and groups you did before your diagnosis, perhaps with some modifications. You may just need to reduce or adapt intensity or modify certain exercises depending on how you're feeling. Pop along to watch a session/group from the side-lines so you can see if it's the right ability level for you and if you like the look of it.

Explain your medical history to the instructor or class leader. They may be nervous or unfamiliar with the implications of your condition, in which case they may find reading this book helps them understand your diagnosis, limitations and needs following bowel cancer. Direct them to the ACSM (American College of Sports Medicine) *Exercise Guidelines for Cancer Survivors*[1] and the Macmillan Cancer Support booklet on *Physical Activity and Cancer*[2] if they have concerns.

If you've had abdominal surgery, it's a good idea to find an instructor who is a specialist in postnatal rehabilitation or who understands the core/pelvic floor/ abdominal pressure issues and how to modify and adapt exercise. Women's health specialists, pre/postnatal instructors and Pilates instructors are often well trained in this area. If you're a man reading this, don't be put off by the 'postnatal' label – the same principles apply. That sort of instructor will be more knowledgeable about your situation.

Home exercise videos/online

The options are endless for home-based exercise. It's a great option for people who are worried about infection or are already immunosuppressed.

Technology now allows us to stream exercise/activity classes straight to our living rooms and you can participate in a class just like you're at the gym. This can be anything from a chair-based yoga-style class to Pilates, weights or a dance class, and the cost per month is usually quite low. There are lots of options – do an online search (and see page 200 for suggestions). Make it simple for yourself by getting your technology, passwords, exercise area and speaker set up so it's easy to log in and workout at a moment's notice.

Some classes and fitness DVDs might not be suitable depending on your condition, complications or stage of diagnosis. Watch the DVD or video all the way through first before you start and then review the 'Precautions and adaptations' in Chapter 3. Modify and adapt any movements or exercises you don't think are suitable.

Macmillan Cancer Support produce a free 'Move More Cancer Exercise' DVD available to order from their website (see page 200). This is a gentle programme which can be done in your living room at home and has a chair-based option. Any postnatal Pilates DVD/video is ideal if you've had abdominal surgery.

Other home exercise

Purchase weights, kettle bells or resistance bands to use at home. Ask a fitness trainer to set you a programme to follow. Work out your own programme of gentle home-based exercises using the exercises in Chapters 7 and 8 of this book and then build from there.

Rent or buy home exercise equipment. Bikes, treadmills, steppers and rowing machines are all available on rental schemes. Use a heartrate monitor to keep the intensity at the right level.

The one downside of home exercise is that it can be hard to be motivated. Your intentions may be good, but there's always something else to do – washing, work, TV, ironing, housework, admin etc soon takes over and always seems more important. Your exercise bike or stack of weights soon start looking dusty! You have to be pretty disciplined to exercise at home, but for some people it can work really well.

Make a pledge

Let's wrap up this chapter – and the book – with some pledges and commitments. We've looked at barriers, benefits and overcoming obstacles, and talked about your support crew. Revisit those mini-exercises at any time.

By committing your pledges to paper, you're more likely to do them. Make three simple pledges to do something to improve your health through activity. It doesn't matter how big or small these pledges are, but they need to be relevant to you and where you are in your cancer recovery journey and to be realistic. In addition to each 'pledge', write down what the benefit will be and what you'll gain from doing it.

Make them specific. Don't just write 'Get more active'. That's too big and non-specific. Instead write 'I pledge to walk at lunchtime for 10 minutes every day'. Keep it realistic and specific so you know you can measure it and tick it off.

Copy these out onto a card and put it somewhere that you'll see every day.

I pledge to:

What will the benefit be?

I pledge to:

What will the benefit be?

I pledge to:

What will the benefit be?

And finally, let's have one last score on the importance and confidence scales.

• How important is it for you to be physically active right now?

1 Not at all important	2	3	4	5	6	7	8	9	10 Extremely important

- How confident do you feel about being physically active right now?

1 Not at all confident	2	3	4	5	6	7	8	9	10 Extremely confident

Compare this with your score right at the beginning of the book in Chapter 1. How does it compare? I really hope you feel more positive, empowered and encouraged to be active, to move a bit more and to find ways to weave movement into your life.

Key points

- Think about what the type of environment you like to be in – don't go to the gym if you love being outdoors in the fresh air.
- If you like music, find a dance class or exercise with a motivating playlist. Or listen to music as you walk or jog.
- Do some research into what's available near you – is there a local cancer exercise class or an exercise referral group at the leisure centre? Try a Nordic walking group, running group or yoga or Pilates class. Many people love Tai Chi, which is great for improving balance.
- What you need to do during cancer and beyond might be very different from what you did before. That's okay. You might go in a new direction. Let the past go and accept that things might be different. Your new mantra is 'flexibility and acceptance'.
- Most of us find it easier to exercise with a friend or group. Find a couple of exercise partners, book sessions with a trainer or ask for a referral to an exercise class from your GP. If you can afford it, book a personal trainer (ideally one who is a trained cancer exercise specialist).
- Ask your family and friends to support and encourage you to be active, to give you a little push on the days when you don't feel like it. It's common for family to worry (and advise you to rest), so perhaps get them to read this book so they feel more confident that what you're doing is safe and good for you.
- Don't leave it to chance. It won't happen unless you make it happen.
- Identify barriers and obstacles that make being active difficult... Identify

what they are and then work out how to break them down. Find ways around obstacles and solutions to difficulties.

- Stay focused on the benefits. Always ask yourself… 'What will I gain from this?' Exercise might not always be fun at the time. No-one bounces out of bed saying, 'Yippee, time for a run!'. Most people find it hard to get going, even when they feel well and are healthy. Sometimes you have to give yourself a little push to get going.
- Always remember that every little bit of movement counts and makes a difference. Every 10-minute walk. Every set of 10 sit-stands. Every time you take the stairs instead of the lift. Every time you do some stretching instead of slumping on the sofa. All of those things make a difference and will help you feel better, get moving and rebuild your confidence.
- Never underestimate the power of movement and physical activity. Something is always better than nothing. And something is always possible. Have the confidence to try.

I'll leave you with this poem. I found it online but cannot find the author. It's wonderful. So, whoever you are who wrote this… thank you!

The more I move, the better I feel
The better I feel, the more I heal
The more I heal, the more I can take
So, let's get moving for goodness sake!

Author unknown

APPENDIX AND REFERENCES

Appendix

My story

I want to share my own personal story with you, as this has been fundamental to my writing this book and has transformed my approach to exercise for myself and my clients.

It was June 2010. I was 36 years old, a fit triathlete and had two small boys. In the middle of the night I woke with agonising abdominal pain. It came from nowhere. I woke my husband who called a doctor. I was rushed to hospital with life-threatening peritonitis due to a perforated colon. I remember lying in hospital saying to the surgeon 'But I'm doing a triathlon in 8 weeks; I'll be better by then, right?' What I didn't realise was that just staying alive was my only goal at that point. Of course, there was no triathlon and what followed was two years of multiple bowel surgeries and ill-health.

I was very poorly and had to have emergency surgery to remove a section of my large bowel. Part of the surgery meant having a stoma (often referred to as a 'colostomy bag' or an ostomy). As explained in Chapter 4, this is a procedure where the end of the small bowel (in my case) is brought to the surface of the skin on the abdomen where the stoma (or ostomy) is formed.

Many people know it as a 'colostomy' or having a 'bag'. Technically it's an ileostomy (the end of the small bowel is called the ileum) and it essentially bypasses the rest of your digestive system and your waste comes out of a hole in your stomach. It's both incredible and weird at the same time.

Back then I'd never heard of an ileostomy, or a stoma, or an ostomy, and didn't know anyone who had one. But I learned fast. It was only meant to be temporary, but there were complications which spanned the following two years. Between 2010 and 2012 I was in and out of hospital countless times and had five major abdominal surgeries. At one stage I thought I would never be able to eat solid food ever again. I was living on liquids and was frail and very poorly. Looking back, I'm not entirely sure how I got through it. I do remember feeling desperately low, desperately ill and at rock bottom. Thankfully, in 2012 I had a successful surgery which meant I got my quality of life back and learned to eat again. My stoma is with me forever now (by my choice) and I'm quite happy about that. I live a normal and very active life and it doesn't really stop me doing anything at all. I am passionate about sharing the message that having a stoma doesn't have to limit your life.

Before being ill I had been fit, healthy and zooming around through life, enjoying competitive sport and being a fitness trainer, coach and health writer. I was busy with my boys and family life and thought I was doing everything right. For me it was a life lesson that none of us are invincible and we have no clue what is round the next corner.

Suddenly I was broken, at rock bottom and had to literally crawl my way back to fitness and health. As an exercise specialist I was naively expecting some kind of 'exercise rehabilitation programme'. But there was nothing. I was left to figure it out on my own. I'd had major abdominal surgery five times, lost two stone in weight (mostly muscle), spent weeks in hospital and was a shadow of my former self. I'd not only lost my fitness, but also my confidence. I didn't know how my body worked and didn't have any belief in it anymore. It had let me down in a big way and I didn't trust it. I felt weak, broken and vulnerable, and I had to learn how to live in a new body, one that had a bag attached to it.

I thought I might just pick up where I'd left off. 'Get back to where I was before' was my mantra. Maybe do a couple of marathons and get back to triathlons. But it wasn't so easy.

After learning to eat again, I had to learn to 'rethink' my relationship with exercise and running, and what it meant to me and what I wanted from my running. I found that I didn't want to be competitive anymore. I had lost the 'pain' button needed to compete at a high level, and I wanted to go in a new direction. I did a competitive 10 km race and hated every minute. Instead, I found that I just wanted to be out in nature, running gently, out on the trail with my husband, without pressure, and with someone who understood what I'd been through. Eight years on we still do marathons, but we do them for the scenery, camaraderie and the cake afterwards. Don't get me wrong, I still like to challenge myself with long-distance running, but it took major surgery and illness to teach me that exercise needed to nourish me and provide comfort.

I've gone on to run multiple marathons (31 at the last count), ultra-distance runs, an incredible 100-mile stage run in the Himalayas in India in 2014 and a 120-mile stage run across the Rockies in Colorado in 2018. But what's been fascinating is that I didn't just 'get back to where I was' – I've gone in a new direction. I'm so much more grateful for good health and being alive, and I have a new-found gratitude for exercise. Running and being able to exercise are a privilege. Not everyone is so lucky. Out of the depths of despair, I've developed a desire to grab life and enjoy every moment I can.

Although at times it was unbearably difficult and I was scared I'd never recover, I tried to see my stoma as just another challenge… something to overcome.

I've always said running is a metaphor for life. It's a roller coaster of difficulty, resilience, fear, happiness, joy and elation. Experiencing illness and surgery is much the same and I've found the skills needed to be a successful runner have helped me overcome challenges with a stoma and vice versa.

So whilst I've not experienced cancer myself, and I'm not presuming to understand how you feel and how your cancer affects you, I've been through my own ordeal. And this experience has taught me empathy and a level of understanding that I wouldn't have had otherwise. It's made me a better trainer and coach and taken me on a new journey into the world of rehabilitation, cancer recovery and clinical exercise.

If you've always been fit, it's impossible to understand just how hard it is when you're sick, weak and vulnerable, dealing with a major illness or surgery. In many ways the cause of the illness or surgery is irrelevant. The roller coaster of treatment, recovery and the aftermath and trauma leaves its mark. You can choose to give in and give up, or you can dig deep and find a way to overcome the challenges and learn to go in a new direction.

About my services

I offer a professional consultancy support service providing 1:1 coaching in person, mentoring or via my 'virtual clinic' on skype/email for anyone with cancer or a stoma. I can offer advice on post-operative exercise, return to fitness, rehabilitation of the abdominal core and safe appropriate exercise during and after cancer treatment and stoma surgery. Find out more about my services at www.sarah-russell.co.uk and my online exercise website www.theostomystudio.co.uk.

Sarah Russell

2019

Scan here to go directly to my website (www.sarah-russell.co.uk).

References and resources

Introduction

References

1. Cancer Research UK. *Bowel cancer statistics*. www.cancerresearchuk.org.uk (accessed 18 August 2021).
2. Clinical Oncology Society of Australia (COSA). *COSA position statement on exercise in cancer care 2018*. www.cosa.org.au/media/332488/cosa-position-statement-v4-web-final.pdf (accessed March 2019).
3. Wolin KY, Yan Y, Colditz GA, Lee IM. Physical activity and colon cancer prevention: a meta-analysis. *British Journal of Cancer* 2009;100(4):611-616.
4. Association of Stoma Care Nurses UK (ASCN). *National Clinical Guidelines 2016*. http://ascnuk.com/wp-content/uploads/2016/03/ASCN-Clinical-Guidelines-Final-25-April-compressed-11-10-38.pdf (accessed 22 March 2019).

Further resources

- McGrattan J. *Sorted: The Active Woman's Guide to Health*. London: Bloomsbury; 2017.
- Dr Lucy Gossage's website: www.cancerfit.me

Chapter 2: Treatments for bowel cancer and how exercise can help

References

1. Macmillan Cancer Support. *Enjoying Life. Physical activity and cancer: the underrated wonder drug.* 2018. www.macmillan.org.uk/_images/physical-activity-and-cancer-the-underrated-wonder-drug_tcm9-336275.pdf (accessed 22 March 2019).

2. Clinical Oncology Society of Australia (COSA). *COSA position statement on exercise in cancer care 2018.* www.cosa.org.au/media/332488/cosa-position-statement-v4-web-final.pdf (accessed March 2019).

3. Wolin KY, Yan Y, Colditz GA, Lee IM. Physical activity and colon cancer prevention: a meta-analysis. *British Journal of Cancer* 2009;100(4):611-616.

4. Cancer Research UK. *What is cancer fatigue?* www.cancerresearchuk.org/about-cancer/coping/physically/fatigue/what-is-cancer-fatigue (accessed 22 March 2019).

5. Stevinson C, Campbell A, Cavill N, Foster J. *Physical Activity and Cancer. A concise evidence review.* Macmillan Cancer Support. 2017. www.macmillan.org.uk/_images/the-importance-physical-activity-for-people-living-with-and-beyond-cancer_tcm9-290123.pdf (accessed 22 March 2019).

6. Evans WJ. Skeletal muscle loss: cachexia, sarcopenia, and inactivity. *The American Journal of Clinical Nutrition* 2010; 91(4):1123S–1127S. http://ajcn.nutrition.org/content/91/4/1123S.full (accessed 22 March 2019).

7. Campbell CS. *Deconditioning: the consequence of bed rest.* Geriatric Research Education Clinical Center. 2011. http://aging.ufl.edu/files/2011/01/deconditioning_campbell.pdf (accessed 22 March 2019).

8. Meyerhardt J, Heseltine D, Niedzwiecki D, Hollis D, Saltz LB, Mayer RJ. Impact of physical activity on cancer recurrence and survival in patients with stage III colon cancer: findings from CALGB 89803. *Journal of Clinical Oncology* 2006; 24(22):3535-3541. https://ascopubs.org/doi/full/10.1200/JCO.2006.06.0863 (accessed 22 March 2019).

Chapter 3: Precautions and adaptations

References

1. Macmillan Cancer Support. *Physical Activity and Cancer*. 2019. 5th Edition. MAC12515_E05_N. http://be.macmillan.org.uk/Downloads/CancerInformation/LivingWithAndAfterCancer/MAC12515E05physical-activitylowresPDF20190128HS.PDF (accessed 22 March 2019).
2. Macmillan Cancer Support. *Physical Activity for People with Metastatic Bone Disease: Guidance for Healthcare Professionals*. www.macmillan.org.uk/_images/physical-activity-for-people-with-metastatic-bone-disease-guidance_tcm9-326004.pdf (accessed 22 March 2019).

Chapter 4: Living and exercising with a stoma

References

1. Bland C, Young K. Nurse activity to prevent and support patients with a parastomal hernia. *Gastrointestinal Nursing* 2015;13(10): 16-24.
2. Association of Stoma Care Nurses UK (ASCN). *National Clinical Guidelines 2016*. http://ascnuk.com/wp-content/uploads/2016/03/ASCN-Clinical-Guidelines-Final-25-April-compressed-11-10-38.pdf (accessed 22 March 2019).
3. Colostomy UK. *Active Ostomates: Sport and Fitness After Stoma Surgery*. May 2018. www.colostomyuk.org/wp-content/uploads/2018/06/Active-Ostomates-Sport-and-fitness-after-stoma-surgery.pdf (accessed 23 March 2019).

Further resources

On behalf of Global medical devices company ConvaTec I developed a specific stoma exercise rehabilitation programme and education package called **me+recovery**. Through this programme we have educated hundreds of nurses and healthcare professionals around the world, including 250 UK stoma nurses. As a patient you can access free resources and information about stoma exercise/rehabilitation, hydration and much more.

If you have a stoma, you can register for more information/resources at www.convatec.co.uk/meplus in the UK or call 0800 467 866.

Stoma further reading

- Russell S. Physical Activity and the stoma patient. Overcoming barriers. *British Journal of Nursing* 2017;26(5):S20–S26.
- McGrath A. Parastomal hernia: an exploration of the risk factors and the implications. *British Journal of Nursing* 2006;15(6): 317-321.
- Thompson M, Trainor B. Incidence of parastomal hernia before and after prevention program. *Gastrointestinal Nursing* 2005; 3(2): 23–7.
- Thompson M, Trainor B. Prevention of parastomal hernia: a comparison of results 3 years on. *Gastrointestinal Nursing* 2007; 5(3): 22–8.

Chapter 5: Fatigue and self-care

References

1. National Cancer Institute. *Fatigue. Patient Version.* June 2017. www.cancer.gov/about-cancer/treatment/side-effects/fatigue/fatigue-pdq (accessed 23 March 2019).
2. Macmillan Cancer Support. *Coping With Fatigue (Tiredness).* 2018. 8th Edition MAC11664_E08. https://www.macmillan.org.uk/_images/MAC11664_E08_Cop_Fatigue_p03_20181105_lowres%20pdf_tcm9-345459.pdf (accessed 23 March 2019).
3. Pemberton S, Berry C. *Fighting Fatigue. A practical guide to managing the symptoms of CFS/ME.* 2009. Hammersmith Books; London, UK.
4. Evans, M. *Cancer Related Fatigue.* Video. Sunnybrook Odette Cancer Centre and the Canadian Cancer Society. http://health.sunnybrook.ca/cancer-fatigue-content/video/ (accessed 23 March 2019).
5. Dweck C. *Mindset. Changing the Way You Think to Fulfil Your Potential.* 6th Edition. Robinson. 2017.
6. National Cancer Institute. *Sleep disorders. Patient version.* 2016. www.cancer.gov/about-cancer/treatment/side-effects/sleep-disorders-pdq (accessed 23 March 2019).
7. Cancer Research UK. *Meditation.* 2015. www.cancerresearchuk.org/about-cancer/cancer-in-general/treatment/complementary-alternative-therapies/individual-therapies/meditation (accessed 23 March 2019).

Further resources

- Untire. This is a free app available for your smartphone especially for people affected with cancer-related fatigue. It has similar tips to Chapter 5 and includes ideas for exercises and daily journaling. See https://untire.me/
- Earplugs: BioEars are a great brand – soft silicone earplugs that you can mould to fit and work really well.
- Sleep trackers. If you like gadgets and data, using a sleep tracker will really appeal. Wearing a tracker as a watch or wristband will give you feedback on the quality and quantity of your sleep, monitoring your heartrate and movement as you sleep. There is a huge choice and the technology and accuracy have improved rapidly in recent years. Just search for 'wearable sleep trackers' online and do some research before you invest. Fitbit seem to lead the way in this area. Data feedback in black and white can be very motivating and can help you identify patterns.
- Meditation apps:
  o Headspace www.headspace.com/
  o Calm: www.calm.com
  o Be Mindful: www.bemindfulonline.com

Chapter 6: Principles of exercise and monitoring

References

1. Department of Health and Social Care. *Start Active, Stay Active. A report on physical activity for health from the four home counties' Chief Medical Officers.* 2011. www.gov.uk/government/publications/start-active-stay-active-a-report-on-physical-activity-from-the-four-home-countries-chief-medical-officers (accessed 23 March 2019).
2. Campbell KL, Winters-Stone KM, Wiskemann J, et al. Exercise Guidelines for Cancer Survivors: Consensus Statement from International Multidisciplinary Roundtable. *Medicine & Science in Sports & Exercise* 2019; 51(11): 2375-2390. doi: 10.1249/MSS.0000000000002116
3. Toohey K, Pumpa K, McKune A, Cooke J, Semple S. High-intensity exercise interventions in cancer survivors: a systematic review exploring the impact on health outcomes. *Journal of Cancer Research and Clinical Oncology* 2018; 144(1): 1-12.

Further resources

- Active 10. A free app for your smartphone that shows you just how briskly (or not) you are walking (www.nhs.uk/oneyou/active10/home)
- Resting heartrate (RHR) app for your phone: www.hrv4training.com
- Fitness tracker watches: Polar (www.polar.com/uk-en) and Fitbit (www.fitbit.com/uk/home)
- Exercise heartrate (HER) chest straps or wrist sensors: Polar; Fitbit or Garmin are usually good brands.

Chapter 7: Core exercises and rehabilitation after surgery

References

1. Association of Stoma Care Nurses UK (ASCN). *National Clinical Guidelines 2016*. http://ascnuk.com/wp-content/uploads/2016/03/ASCN-Clinical-Guidelines-Final-25-April-compressed-11-10-38.pdf (accessed 22 March 2019).

Further resources

- Pelvic floor exercise app: NHS Squeezy App (www.squeezyapp.co.uk). This inexpensive app is a brilliant tool which you can personalise and use to set reminders on your phone to do your pelvic floor exercises throughout the day.
- Step counter apps: Active 10 (www.nhs.uk/oneyou/active10/home); Fitbit.

Abdominal exercises and pelvic floor resources

- Pelvic Obstetric & Gynaecological Physiotherapy. *Fit Following Surgery: Advice and Exercise Following Major Gynaecological Surgery*. 2017. https://pogp.csp.org.uk/publications/fit-following-surgery-advice-and-exercise-following-major-gynaecological-surgery (accessed 23 March 2019).
- Pelvic Exercises, an online resource created by Michelle Kenway to provide women with information about pelvic floor problems.
    - o   *Safe Exercises After a Hysterectomy – Health Professional Guidelines*. www.pelvicexercises.com.au/hyster-exercise-guidelines/ (accessed 23 March 2019).

o   *Inside Out: Pelvic Floor Safe Exercise Book.*
    www.pelvicexercises.com.au/pelvic-exercise-products/pelvic-
    exercise-books/inside-out-michelle-kenway/

- Birmingham Bowel Clinic. *Colostomy and Exercise.* 2014.
  www.birminghambowelclinic.co.uk/files/20140521164955-Colostomy-and-
  Exercise.pdf
- Continence Association of Australia – Excellent resources
  www.continence.org.au
- Sue Croft – Australian Physiotherapist with special interest in continence and
  pelvic floor health. Superb resources and great books:
  www.suecroftphysiotherapist.com.au
- Diane Lee – https://dianelee.ca/article-training-deep-core-muscles.php

Chapter 9: Diet and lifestyle

References

1. World Cancer Research Fund. *Cancer Prevention Recommendations.*
    www.wcrf.org/dietandcancer/cancer-prevention-recommendations (accessed
    23 March 2019).
2. Kastorini C-M, Milionis HJ, Esposito K, Giugliano D, Goudevenos JA,
    Panagiotakos DB. The effect of Mediterranean diet on metabolic syndrome
    and its components: a meta-analysis of 50 studies and 534,906 individuals.
    Journal of the American College of Cardiology 2011; 57(11):1299-1313.
3. Cancer Research UK. *The Microbiome and Cancer: What's All the Fuss
    About?* 2017. www.cancerresearchuk.org/funding-for-researchers/research-
    features/2017-06-13-the-microbiome-and-cancer-whats-all-the-fuss-about
    (accessed 23 March 2019).
4. WCRF. *Eat Well During Cancer.* www.wcrf-uk.org/uk/here-help/eat-well-
    during-cancer (accessed 23 March 2019).
5. National Cancer Institute. *Eating Hints – Before, During and After Cancer
    Treatment.* www.cancer.gov/publications/patient-education/eatinghints.pdf
    (accessed 23 March 2019).

Further resources

- Protein whey isolate powder supplement: www.pulsin.co.uk
- BEAT – the charity for eating disorders: www.beateatingdisorders.org.uk
- Electrolyte drinks: Dioralyte (www.dioralyte.co.uk);
  SOS Rehydrate (www.sosrehydrate.com).

Chapter 10: Overcoming barriers and getting motivated

References

1. Schmitz KH, Courneya KS, Matthews C, Denmark-Wahnefried W, Galvao DA, Pinto BM, Irwin ML, Wolin KY, Segal RJ, Lucia A, Schneider CM, von Gruenigen VE, Schwartz AL. American College of Sports Medicine roundtable on exercise guidelines for cancer survivors. *Medical Science of Sports Exercise* 2010l;42(7):1409-26.
2. Macmillan Cancer Support. *Physical Activity and Cancer*. January 2019. 5th Edition. MAC12515_E05_N. http://be.macmillan.org.uk/Downloads/CancerInformation/LivingWithAndAfterCancer/MAC12515E05physical-activitylowresPDF20190128HS.PDF

Further resources

- Online activity videos: Pilatesanytime.com
- Macmillan Cancer Support: Move More DVD (https://be.macmillan.org.uk/be/p-20843-move-more-dvd.aspx)

Index